Pelican Book A819

Studies in Social Pathology

Editor: G. M. Carstairs

VENEREAL DISEASES

Dr R. S. Morton was educated in Glasgow and qualified there in medicine in 1939. He spent six years with the Royal Army Medical Corps in the Middle East and Europe and was awarded the M.B.E.

On his return from the war he decided to make a career in venereology, trained at Newcastle upon Tyne and took his specialist qualification in Edinburgh. For nine years he held a consultant post in Cheshire and then Manchester, until in 1960 he was appointed consultant to the Sheffield area. He is lecturer and clinical tutor in venereal diseases in Sheffield University and its associated teaching hospitals and is active in the various national committees concerned with his speciality.

Dr Morton has published many studies on problems in venereology. The epidemiology, the social background and the prevention of venereal diseases have especially concerned him. He is married with two sons.

R. S. Morton

Venereal Diseases

The best prophet of the future is the past – *Byron*

Prosperity doth best discover Vice – *Bacon*

 Penguin Books

Penguin Books Ltd, Harmondsworth, Middlesex, England
Penguin Books Inc., 3300 Clipper Mill Road, Baltimore 11, Md, U.S.A.
Penguin Books Pty Ltd, Ringwood, Victoria, Australia

First published 1966
Copyright © R. S. Morton, 1966

Made and printed in Great Britain by
Cox & Wyman Ltd,
London, Fakenham and Reading
Set in Monotype Times

Contents

Editorial Foreword 7

Preface 9

Acknowledgements 11

1. Feelings and Fact 13

2. Venereal Diseases Yesterday 19

3. Venereal Diseases Today 33

4. Principally about Gonorrhoea 50

5. Principally about Syphilis 67

6. Principally about Other Sexually Transmitted
   Diseases 91

7. Venereal Diseases as a Social Problem 112

8. Venereal Diseases as a Medical Problem 134

9. Variations on an Enigma 162
   References 175
   Index 183

Editorial Foreword

In primitive societies, most diseases (together with all other inexplicable misfortunes) are thought to be due to the action of hostile or angry spirits. Their victims enlist the help of shamans to discover what action on their part has offended the gods, and what must be done to propitiate them. This is especially true of certain more than usually dreaded conditions, such as smallpox or leprosy. In India, for example, one can still find communities where it is believed that leprosy is a visitation upon the children of one who has committed the supreme impiety, in Hindu eyes, of causing the death of a cow. It is only gradually, over many centuries, that sick people have learned that they do not need to feel guilty, as well as feeling ill. Many of us can well remember the shame which used until quite recently be attached to families which were 'tainted' with tuberculosis: that particular source of shame has melted away with the discovery of a radical cure for this infection.

The same cannot be said for venereal disease. In our society, though not in some others, venereal disease is still regarded as a shameful condition, a moral as well as a physical degradation. Not many years ago these feelings were held much more strongly, particularly by the more sanctimonious. Many pious people believed that pain and suffering were the just retribution of transgression; and since venereal disease was commonly associated with violations of sexual morality, its victims received little consideration. During the early decades of the

Editorial Foreword.

century the treatment of syphilis and gonorrhoea was often painful and seldom very effective: but since the mid nineteen-forties, penicillin has transformed the situation. Now both these illnesses, if treated early, can be cured quickly and painlessly. If it were not for a third, more intractable condition (non-specific urethritis), moralists might soon be confronted with the alarming prospect of a world in which sexual promiscuity was freed of its age-long attendant threat of disease.

Moralistic attitudes have continued to be attached to these diseases even after the discovery of their cause, because the behaviour which perpetuates their spread is socially disapproved. It has long been known that venereal diseases are most rife in those sections of society which betray other indices of social disorganization, in areas of poverty and overcrowding, where there are high rates of delinquency and crime, of broken homes, marital disharmony, drunkenness and attempted suicide. Clearly, therefore, venereal disease is as much a social as it is a medical problem.

It is in this light that Dr Morton has approached his subject, paying attention to its social history and its social psychology as well as giving a clear, factual account of present medical knowledge about venereal disease. When he discusses treatment, also, this is viewed not only from the point of view of curative and preventive medicine, but also as an application of social policy which must be grounded in the science of human behaviour. This is a dispassionate study of a theme which has often aroused strong emotions; but the level-headed assessments and remedies which it offers reveal a very practical compassion.

G. M. CARSTAIRS

Preface

This book is descriptive. It does not tell a pretty story. It is quite unsuited to those who, even theoretically, have not equipped themselves with an understanding of human sex. Indeed those who cannot appreciate what sex means in terms of joy, or misery, fulfilment, or frustration, happy marriage and social disaster (and this must include many young people), will find little in it. Grown-ups with rigid personalities, rooted in blind authoritarianism, unbending prudery, religion or solid prejudice likewise will find it disappointing if not infuriating. It will make the libertine unhappy.

Those prone to hypochondriacal introspection about their mental or bodily functions will do well to avoid it.

Those seeking a merry tale or two of sexual adventure will find none.

The book is an attempt to present soberly and factually a full account of the venereal and other sexually transmitted diseases. It is for those who find the urge for knowledge satisfied in its pursuit and for those to whom the study of man's behaviour evokes perpetual wonder.

Doctors are sometimes accused of living and working in a vacuum, concerning themselves only with individuals and all too little with social awareness or purpose. Those who choose to stand back for a moment to look at the wood rather than the individual trees risk being accused of 'under-selling' medicine, precipitating unnecessary anxiety or of 'empire-building'. I have taken such risks sure in the belief that a view of the wood will be found to dominate the social scene and its future more that any single tree in it.

Acknowledgements

I am indebted to Mr A. S. Foster, Medical Artist to United Sheffield Hospitals, for preparing and supplying all the illustrations.

My cordial thanks are due to Dr S. M. Laird for his encouragement and helpful criticism and to Dr G. S. Andrew for reading the proofs.

1   Feelings and Fact

Our feelings are often strangely mixed when we find ourselves in the presence of someone physically or mentally maimed by accident or disease. We are aware of simultaneous compassion and revulsion or even pity with disgust. The reality of the victim's plight and such opposing emotions, however, we can usually accept with relative calm. This is less likely to be the experience of some people when the confrontation is with an infectious condition. Compassion may be swamped by outright repugnance and pity shrinks in the presence of alarm. This is certainly so with the venereal diseases. The responses evoked by close contact with these are frequently extreme.

When, for example, a factory-worker's fellows learn that he or she has 'V.D.' the news spreads rapidly. The contagiousness of the condition is liable to be magnified. Everything the victim has touched is rumoured to be fouled. Demands are made on the management for the victim's removal. The works lavatories are declared unusable. Threats of strike action may follow. Common sense is challenged and over-run. Emotions crystallize in a threatening communal synthesis. Such situations are not uncommon even today. In the span of four years aid was sought from the author in the settlement of three such upheavals. In one, the victim, a laundry worker, did not have, and never had had, venereal infection. Vicious and hostile feelings prevailed in these circumstances. The vehemence of both men and women was intense and their condemnation often vitriolic. 'Lock him up', 'Whip her', 'Lack of moral fibre', 'Dirty bitch', 'Force him to have treatment', 'Sack her'. There is no ambivalence here: no hint of compassion, pity or even humility. We can only sense, beneath the heat, the smugly satisfying glow of self-righteousness and wonder at the near-hysterical demands for ostracism.

It is perhaps some comfort to recognize that, vicious as these blind reactions may be, they show some advance in civilization and sophistication from reactions in 1497. At that time, when syphilis was rife in Europe, an Act was passed in Edinburgh ordering all those infected to assemble on the sands of Leith, by 10 a.m. on a Friday morning, whence they would be taken by boat to the offshore island of Inchkeith. The whole operation was to be completed by sunset on the following Monday. Failure to comply was to be punished by branding on the cheek so that sufferers 'may be kennit in time to come'.

Another attitude, quite different, more widespread and no less alarming, prevails about venereal disease. This is one of comfortable detachment. The reasoning, if such it can be called, goes something like this: 'I have never had it, I have never known anybody have it, therefore either it doesn't exist or is very, very rare. If it occurs at all then it happens only to loose women, the poor, soldiers, or the people who never wash.' In contrast to the first and aggressive type of reaction, where V.D. was outrageously over-emphasized, here it is played down to the level of being unrecognized. It is true that venereal diseases are seldom recognizably obvious. There is no way of knowing, for example, whether the man opposite you in the train is under treatment for syphilis. The hidden nature of much sexually transmitted disease is certainly not obvious in the demeanour of a cheerful young woman only recently named as a source of gonorrhoea. One doesn't hear a man relate his anguish at discovering signs of infection or a woman recall her sense of outraged pride when asked by her husband to seek advice about the gonorrhoea he has passed to her. Such omissions nurture detachment.

The basis of these two different attitudes to venereal disease – the hostile and the repressed – is of course emotional and born of ignorance and rationalization. The facts do not vary. For a rational understanding of them we must concern ourselves with definitions, terminology, prevalence rates, historical background and the clinical course and natural history of the diseases. We will look to where and how the diseases are dealt with and the medical and epidemiological problems involved. We will try to gain some understanding of the individual and social circumstances associated with rises and falls of incidence. In other words, we will attempt an ecological appraisal. Not least, we will try to view our own national position against the world background.

In *Through the Looking Glass*, Alice at one time found herself sorely tried by a schizoid conversation with Humpty Dumpty.

'There's glory for you.'

'I don't know what you mean by "glory",' Alice said.

'I meant "there's a nice knock-down argument for you!"'

'But "glory" doesn't mean "a nice knock-down argument",' Alice objected.

'When *I* use a word,' Humpty Dumpty said in rather a scornful tone, 'it means just what I choose it to mean – neither more nor less.'

The adjective 'venereal' means that the infections so named are communicated from one person to another by and during sexual intercourse or contact. (The sexual activity may be hetero- or homosexual.) Venereal diseases are therefore sexually transmitted. There are some well-recognized and comparatively rare exceptions to the sex-transmission rule. Some children and adults are born with syphilis, being infected in the womb by their mothers. Syphilis has been reported after transfusions of fresh blood and after tattooing. Babies may suffer gonococcal eye infection by contamination with their mothers' discharge at birth. Spread by non-sexual contact, i.e. by simply touching, is very, very rare. Contrary to some peoples' belief, spread by contact with such things as lavatory seats, cricket balls and camel bites is unknown. Venereal diseases or other sexually transmitted diseases have nothing to do with poverty, dirt, lack of sanitation or personal hygiene *per se*. They cannot be self-engendered. They do not arise spontaneously even in the most socially unacceptable places or people.

Of about a dozen diseases capable of being spread during

intercourse, only three, gonorrhoea, syphilis and chancroid, are defined in law as venereal. (There is no division in the medical mind between venereal and sexually transmitted diseases.) Gonorrhoea, by far the commonest, is an infection beginning in and usually confined to the linings of the generative and urinary organs. Characteristically, it gives rise in men to a discharge of pus or matter from the penis (urethritis). In women infection with gonorrhoea is usually without symptoms until complications have arisen. Syphilis, although less common, is the more deadly disease. For the first few months or years it presents as an infection of body surfaces, such as skin and lining of the mouth and throat. Even in the early stages it invades many if not all organs of the body. This stage is followed by a period, varying from five to fifty years, when the disease lies dormant in the body's tissues or organs. Thereafter, and in a proportion of cases only, syphilis manifests itself again in forms which are sometimes disfiguring, sometimes chronically crippling and sometimes deadly. Syphilitic expectant mothers may infect their unborn children, as we shall see later.

Chancroid, or soft sore, is an acute, painful, ulcerative condition of the genitals, more commonly seen in men and more common in tropical and sub-tropical areas of the world than in the more temperate zones.

The great mass of all venereal disease is gonorrhoea and syphilis, and these two infections pose the essential public health problem. They are widely documented and the best understood of all sexually transmitted diseases. From a factual point of view they will therefore play a large part in our discussion. They are not, however, as mention of chancroid suggests, the only part of the problem.

Lymphogranuloma venereum, which is caused by a virus, is more common in para-tropical countries. This disease is occasionally imported into the United Kingdom, to give rise to evanescent genital sores and marked gland enlargements in the groin and in the pelvis of its victims. Granuloma inguinale, or Donovaniasis, yet another type of infection, is now a very rare sexually acquired disease in any part of the world.

Twenty-five years ago our list would have all but ended here. Since the end of the last war, however, there has been increasing evidence that a high proportion of cases of two other common conditions is sexually transmitted.

The first of these is non-specific urethritis, a disease affecting the lining of the male urethra – that canal which passes through a man's penis from the bladder, or urine reservoir, to the exterior. The condition, as recognized at present, is confined to men. (No associated, clearly defined collection of symptoms or signs is so far recognized as occurring in women.) In clinical appearance non-specific urethritis in men is often very like gonorrhoea. By 'non-specific' is meant that no specific and discernible bacterial, viral, protozoal, allergic or chemical cause has yet been found to explain the condition. Nevertheless there is increasing support for the idea that the condition in men is a viral infection, usually acquired during sexual intercourse. Non-specific urethritis is the commonest of all forms of non-gonococcal urethritis.

The second common condition, recognized as frequently sexually transmitted, is infestation by the protozoan or one-celled microscopic animal, called the trichomonas vaginalis. There is a subtle difference in the medical mind between infection and infestation. The former is usually any condition caused by bacteria or viruses. These usually penetrate the superficial layers of a body surface, external or internal, and from such a bridgehead may invade other organs. An infestation, on the other hand, is a condition caused by a parasite of a size larger than a virus or bacterium. Such parasites live on, rather than in, the surfaces of the body or one of its cavities; lice, for example, live on the skin, worms in the bowel. In the present instance we are concerned with infestation of the vagina. The trichomonas vaginalis is the commonest cause of pathological vaginal discharge and is well recognized as one of the causes of urethritis in men. The term trichomoniasis is often used for the disease.

Other conditions, such as the skin diseases of scabies (sometimes called 'the itch'), genital warts and infestation by lice may be acquired during sexual intercourse or while sharing a bed with an infested person.

Such then in brief are the commonest sexually transmitted diseases. Their spread has continued day by day, man to woman, year by year, woman to man (sometimes man to man), decade by decade, one generation to the next throughout the centuries and over the face of the earth.

A look at the history of the best known of the diseases concerned comprises an essential part of our understanding. Indeed, a backward look is imperative for a full appreciation of present problems; and a necessity, too, if we are to estimate, with any confidence or benefit, the prospects and needs of the future.

2   Venereal Diseases Yesterday

Historically, the venereal diseases are proving one of the most difficult of all medico-social problems to unravel. The term 'venereal disease' was introduced by Jacques de Bethercourt in 1527. From some time near this date till the end of the eighteenth and beginning of the nineteenth centuries the term is used in the singular, for gonorrhoea and syphilis were considered to be one and the same disease. History was, in a way, to repeat itself. Many cases of urethritis in men, in which the causative organism was not found, were believed, until about two decades ago, to be gonococcal. It was not until the advent of penicillin, which dealt so effectively with gonococcal urethritis, that non-specific urethritis became recognized as a separate clinical entity. The term 'sexually transmitted diseases' is of recent origin. The histories of these conditions are brief, well documented and devoid of speculation or glamour. Details will be found with the description of these diseases.

The history of syphilis has proved of compelling fascination to medical historians. Knowledge of it dates from the great European epidemic of 1495 onwards, but it is the much earlier recognized disease of gonorrhoea with which we will deal first.

Biblical sources are quoted to substantiate that gonorrhoea plagued man from earliest times. In Leviticus xv we read that when a man has an 'issue' (interpreted as a urethral discharge) he is unclean. It is clear from the descriptions that he is so 'unclean' as to be infectious by contact. The need for washing after copulation is recognized. Moses, the first thorough-going public health administrator, gave very clear orders about the prevention of spread of disease. In Numbers xxxi we learn that the 12,000 Israelites, making war on the Midianites, are held outside the city for seven days after their return to allow for incubation of any disease and subsequent isolation for treatment. All the Midianite women prisoners, 'that have known man by lying with him', were ordered to be killed, to prevent 'a plague among the congregation'. Such extreme measures for the care of the public health are not currently in use anywhere. From other old manuscripts little can be learned about gonorrhoea. It has frequently been remarked upon, and found a source of great surprise, that nothing clearly definitive of the condition is to be found in the classical writings, medical or otherwise, of Greece or Rome.

The first we hear of the disease in this country is in a London Act of 1161, which forbade the brothel keepers of Southwark to house 'women suffering from the perilous infirmity of burning'. The early English terms of 'burning' or 'brenning' are in keeping with the old French name of '*la chaude pisse*', imported probably by the Normans. The word 'burning' is first coupled with the name 'clap' for gonorrhoea in a manuscript by one John of Arderne in 1378. The origin of this colourful but now obsolete word 'clap' is not at all clear. It probably comes from an old French word 'clapoir' meaning 'bosse, bubo or panus inginis', according to the Oxford Dictionary. Yet another term for the condition can be found in a London order of 1430, designed to prohibit brothel keepers from admitting men suffering from '*infirmitas nefanda*' – the hidden disease. The recognition, in these regulations, of the part played by sex, is really quite remarkable, as in the dark ages all diseases were believed to stem from supernatural causes or, later, to be the result of earthquakes, comets or at best the 'miasmas' or emanations of air pollution. Enlightenment came only with the Renaissance. Even then all had to be learned on the basis of father-to-son and teacher-to-pupil. Doubtlessly omissions, alterations and secondary elaborations took place. In the absence of records it is perhaps little wonder that gonorrhoea and syphilis should, following the appearance of syphilis in 1495, be thought to be one and the same condition.

In the eighteenth century in England, at a time when, according to a book entitled *The Laws of Chance* (1738), 'It is hardly one in ten that a Town Spark of that age has not been clapt', the belief of a single 'venereal disease' persisted. Indeed it was 'proved' by the renowned Scottish surgeon, in London, John Hunter (1728–93). He believed that much depended on the site of inoculation of the 'poison' whether the ensuing condition presented as a urethral discharge or an ulcer of the genitals. Unfortunately for him, for countless thousands more, and no less for medical progress – he held up the differentiation of the two diseases for more than half a century – Hunter inoculated himself from a patient who had both syphilis and gonorrhoea. His syphilis, so foolhardily acquired, contributed to the crippling illness of his later life and eventually to his death.

In 1793 Benjamin Bell, of Edinburgh, was the first to separate the two conditions. More cautious than Hunter, he inoculated his students. William Wallace of Dublin, to prove that the rash of syphilis, as well as the initial genital ulcer, was contagious, showed caution if not kindness. He inoculated healthy patients. All these findings were confirmed in Paris by Philipe Ricord, then the doyen of continental venereology.

It was not until 1879 that the diagnosis of gonorrhoea was placed on a scientific basis. In that year the causal organism was identified. Six years later it could be grown and fulfil the essential criterion of producing the disease on experimental inoculation of the human subject.

Until the mid-1930s the treatment of gonorrhoea was by local washes, so-called curative vaccines or very weak antiseptics taken by mouth and excreted in the urine. The doctors' repertoire was very restricted. With the introduction of the sulphonamides in the late 1930s gonorrhoea therapy first reached a scientific level. Success, however, was short-lived. In less than a decade the efficacy of these drugs waned, till they offered hope to a very modest percentage of sufferers only. For the majority, the old-fashioned measures were renewed and the old familiar

complications were common. The dramatic turn of events
effected by the timely arrival of penicillin in 1943 is exemplified
by the outcome of the situation which confronted venereologists
with the British Army in Italy in that year. Many hundreds of
hospital beds were occupied by servicemen with infectious
gonorrhoea. Many cases were complicated. Sulphonamides had
failed with all of them. It was a courageous decision to make the
new wonder drug, as yet manufactured in only small quantities,
available. Within some three weeks almost all the men concerned had returned to their units, cured.

There are two schools of thought on the origin of syphilis –
the Unitarian or Unionist, and the Columbian. The Unitarians
or Unionists believe that there are many diseases in the world
which are in fact one and the same disease, altered only by social
conditions, personal habits and climate. This disease the Unitarians call treponematosis. Syphilis, say the Unitarians, is but
one form of it.

The Columbian school on the other hand believes that the
disease of syphilis did not exist in Europe or the East until
Columbus and his men returned with it from their voyage of
discovery of the Americas in March 1493. Syphilis, this theory
holds, is distinct and different from some other forms of treponematoses, but related.

Although there may be dispute about which of these two
theories is the correct one, all historians are agreed that a
virulent epidemic of the disease which we know as syphilis raged
in Europe from the end of the fifteenth century to the middle of
the sixteenth. The first description was published in 1497 by a
Portuguese physician who worked in Barcelona. He was Ruy
Diaz de Isla (1462–1542) and he claimed to have treated some of
Columbus's men for what they called 'Indian measles'. He
spoke of it as 'a disease, previously unknown, unseen and un-
described which first appeared in that city [Barcelona] . . . and
spread thence throughout the world'.

The infection next appeared among the troops of both sides
during the siege of Naples in 1495. Charles VIII of France invaded Italy about this time. His army consisted largely of

European mercenaries and there were supporting elements such as French artisans and German technicians as well as some 800 camp followers. Spanish soldiers, many recently arrived from their homeland to help defend Naples, were withdrawn on the approach of Charles's army, but not apparently before there had been time for them to infect many of the local women.

There was no great battle, and the infected women of Naples met the French Army with open arms. By way of returning the compliment the Neapolitan men, now themselves infected, left ample reservoirs of disease in the 800 prostitutes of the French camp. No sooner was the encounter over than Charles paid and dispersed his troops, each man free to make his way through Europe to his own country. As a consequence, infection spread like wildfire. Each country blamed its neighbour. The French called it the 'Italian disease', the Germans blamed the French, calling it 'Malade Frantzos'. The English called it the 'French pox'. Spread to the East from Europe is credited to Vasco da Gama and other Portuguese navigators. We learn of the disease in India as early as 1498 and in Canton seven years later. The Japanese word 'mankabassam', i.e. syphilis, means literally, 'the Portuguese sickness'.

Detailed study of the invasion by syphilis of an individual country is rare.

The spread to Scotland, however, has been detailed and is ascribed to the followers of Perkin Warbeck, who pretended to be the Duke of York, the younger of the two princes murdered in the Tower.[76] Warbeck sought the help of James IV of Scotland and, through the support he received, was able to invade England from the north in September 1496. His 1,400 followers consisted of 'some bankrupt, some false English sanctuary men, some thieves, robbers and vagabonds, which leaving their bodily labours, desiring only to live of robbery and raping, became his servants and soldiers'.

Old records of Aberdeen show that eight of Warbeck's supporters preceded him to Scotland and were billeted locally. They were part of that motley crew of 'valiant Captains of all nations' who had travelled from the continent. Who knows but

that some may have served Charles VIII at Naples. The first of
Warbeck's men arrived in Aberdeen in August 1495. They left
in July 1497, three months after the publication by the burgh
authorities of a regulation which clearly recognized the venereal
element in the spread of the new disease. The regulations called
for 'all light [loose] women to decist from their vice and syne of
venerie' and to work for their own support on pain of being
branded. By 1507 the Aberdonians were truly alarmed. A
second regulation exhorted 'that diligent inquisition be taken of
ale infect personnis with this strange sickness of Napillis for the
sautie [safety] of the toun'. The infected were advised to 'keip
quyat in their houssis'.

Similar edicts were being issued in various parts of Europe.
There is no doubt that the disease was new to the doctors and
this gives support to the Columbian theory. Further support
comes from the fact that nowhere in Europe have pre-
Columbian bones been found showing unequivocal evidence of
syphilis. Such bones are claimed to have been found in the
Americas. Another point cited is that nothing at all in the way
of undoubted evidence of syphilis is found in the richly detailed
writings of the early civilizations of the eastern Mediterranean.

The Unitarian or Unionist school of thought views syphilis as
simply one form of a single disease called treponematosis. This
disease is seen most commonly as sub-tropical and spread by
social, rather than sexual contact. It is noted as specially
prevalent among children in poor social and unhygienic conditions. The clinical manifestations of the common form of
the disease vary with race and climate, especially climate. The
commonest forms are yaws, occurring in hot and humid areas of
the world, pinta in South America, and bejel in the hot dry
deserts, notably those of the valley of the Euphrates river. These
are the common tropical and sub-tropical varieties. All start
with a primary ulcer – in yaws, called a 'mother' yaw – followed
by widespread and randomly scattered swellings ('daughter'
yaws) which in the warm, moist atmosphere are luxuriant,
raspberry-like lesions. Bejel of the deserts, however, gives small,

dry crusted lesions. Pinta lesions fall between these two descriptions in appearance and tend to be associated with areas of severe pigmentation and depigmentation. Unlike venereal syphilis all other forms of treponematosis are not potential killers. Nor do they cause pre-natal infection.

Other forms of treponematosis are known as endemic syphilis and occur in temperate zones. One has recently been eradicated from Bosnia in south-eastern Europe. This form was recognized as a social contact disease even in adults, although it was thought by some to be capable of sexual spread. Such endemic and social contact forms of treponematosis are generally associated with poor living conditions. Some of them have died out with the spread of civilization; for example, witkop in South Africa, boomerang leg in Australia and radesgye in Scandinavia. During the seventeenth and eighteenth centuries similar forms existed in the British Isles and Canada. Of particular interest is the button scurvy of Ireland and the sibbens or sivvens of Scotland. Lest any Englishman places undue emphasis on the part played by poor social conditions in the spread of these diseases, it should be pointed out that sibbens was said to have been introduced into Scotland by Cromwell's army. Not unnaturally, and somewhat graciously, his soldiers knew it as the 'Scotch pox'.

The Unitarian theory sees venereal syphilis as but one form of treponematosis. It visualizes the causal organism as, baffled by improving hygiene, clothes and a cold climate, resorting to spread by the only form of bodily contact left to it, that is, sexual contact or intercourse.

According to Hudson,[47] who has laid an increasing load of evidence and theorizing in favour of the Unitarian view, treponematosis started millions of years ago in equatorial Africa with primitive man. As man developed and the original slave trade expanded from central Africa to the north and east, so the disease was spread, altering its appearance with place, race and weather conditions.

Biblical instances are cited in support by some. Syphilis is said to be a possible explanation for the disease which led to the death of 24,000 worshippers of Baal Peor after whoredom with the daughters of Maob (Numbers xxv). There is also the story of the botch of Egypt reported in Deuteronomy xxviii. However, claims that bones, dating from the days of ancient Egypt, show evidence consistent with treponemal disease are not credited with real authority. Lancerveux, in his treatise on syphilis dated 1868, quotes instances from ancient Chinese and Indian sources and also from the writings of the earliest physicians, Hippocrates, Celsus, Galen and Martial, in support of the Unitarian view. Such quotations are generally considered thoroughly inconclusive.

The Unitarian theory seeks to explain the European epidemic in one of two ways. Firstly, the disease could have existed in some mild form in Europe for centuries, the organism suddenly developing a new and deadly virulence.[42] Alternatively, the epidemic stemmed from an alteration in the organism of yaws, when that disease was introduced from West Africa via Portugal in the half-century before Columbus's voyages. Another possibility is that yaws might have been particularly virulent to medieval Europeans, especially as they had no natural resistance to it. Certainly the Unitarian theory is all-embracing. It explains why the diseases are caused by an identical organism which effects identical changes in the blood. Thus while its supporters talk of *Treponematosis*, the Columbians, with their eyes on the very different clinical appearances of the treponemal diseases, talk of *Treponematoses*.

Among the many dozens of names accorded to venereal syphilis in the beginning, one of the most lasting has been 'the pox'. This began as 'the great pox', presumably to distinguish it from the small and chicken varieties. The term 'pox', which more generally means a sore or scar, survived in its original meaning at least till Regency times, when Brummell-like dandies, wishing to give satirical emphasis to condemnation of a colleague, did not only cry 'A plague on you, Sir,' but specified that the plague be 'a pox'. It was clear that they hoped their rivals' amours would founder in infection.

The name 'syphilis' arises from a Latin poem, written in 1530 by a physician, Fracastorius. He wrote several books on contagious diseases and he took the method of poetry to bring home to people the sexual origin of this disease. Syphilis was the name of his shepherd hero who 'became smitten because he raised forbidden altars on the hill'.

Tens of thousands died in the hundred years or so of the European epidemic. There are sound clinical descriptions by the physician Astruc[2] who collected and catalogued all the available descriptions of the earliest writers. There is no doubt that the disease baffled the doctors by its newness and its virulence. Its severity waned, however, over more than a century. Astruc, tracing the epidemic's decline, fixed five periods to the process. Those affected in the first years had widespread rashes, often ulcerative and extending into the mouth and nose to affect the palate and throat. Bone pains and fever were common. In the middle period the rash was less prominent, but tumours filled with gummy material were a predominant feature. Baldness and loss of teeth were common. Bony pains, especially at night, were still a feature in the late years. By 1610 the early disease was more as we see it today – a severe infection but unlikely to kill. The last recorded death from early infectious syphilis in this country was in Leeds some fifteen years ago.

This takes us to a consideration of treatment. At first, only prayer seems to have been available. The emergency, created by the outbreak, led to calling into service one of the Church's fourteen emergency-duty saints. So it was that St Denis became the patron saint of syphilitics. That he is also patron saint of France and Paris is noteworthy. Of all the names accorded to the disease in its earliest years, those referring to its French origin predominated. A short prayer of intercession to St Denis, printed in black and white from a woodcut by Georg Stucks of Nuremberg, was available for sale in 1497. One such, delightfully painted, is held by the Bavarian State Library in Munich. In it, St Denis appears with the Virgin, as do all emergency saints in such printed prayers. At each bottom corner a pock-marked penitent kneels, with head upturned in intercession.

Mercury, in ointment form, long used for skin diseases and known throughout Europe and the Near East from the days of the Crusaders, was widely employed. It was most effective against syphilis. Care had to be taken, as over-use led to the loss of teeth and kidney complications. Alternative methods of employing it were used as the decades went by. Instead of the ointment 'rubs', oral preparations and fumigations were employed. One ingenious artist, finding all such methods unsavoury, rubbed the ointment into his goat, with whom he shared the customary attic, and claimed to cure himself by drinking the animal's milk. For more than four hundred years mercury remained the only remedy of any lasting value. Among many drugs which enjoyed a short spell of popularity was guaiacum, a drug extracted from the resin of lignum vitae, obtained from the West Indies. Its use was strongly advocated by a family who had made a corner in the imports. It is not therefore surprising that guaiacum fell into disuse before long.

At the beginning of the nineteenth century William Wallace, of Dublin, introduced potassium iodide in the treatment of syphilis. Even today it is occasionally employed in conjunction with modern therapy in just the very type of case for which Wallace originally recommended it.

As the nineteenth century advanced, the late manifestations of syphilis came to be definitely associated with earlier forms of the disease. Tabes dorsalis, a variety of paralysis of the legs, and general paralysis of the insane, or syphilitic insanity, were recognized as part and parcel of the illness.

This century's contributions have included discovery of the causative organism – the treponema pallidum – in 1905, the introduction of diagnostic blood tests in 1906, the discovery of suitable and curative arsenical preparations as from 1909, the employment of penicillin in 1943, and most recently, the discovery of a new and highly specific blood test for the diagnosis, or exclusion, of syphilis in dealing with problem cases.

Little can be said about the history of the other form of venereal disease.

Chancroid long continued to be confused and classed as a form of syphilis, at least until the causative organism was discovered in 1889. In the belief that syphilis and chancroid were one and the same disease. Aurias-Turenne in the 1800s recommended repeated re-inoculations with pus from each fresh soft sore produced. By such 'syphilization' he offered protection, shortening of treatment and the avoidance of re-infection or relapse. Aurias-Turenne's methods were tried out in London without success. After his death in 1878 it was found that his body was covered in scars from experiments on himself, yet another example of how blind faith can be a threat to advance.

But what of the social views and aspects of the venereal diseases? The Restoration followed Cromwell's Commonwealth in much the same way as the present has followed Victorianism. In each instance, it is said, a period of strict discipline and puritanism is followed by one of permissiveness. The Restoration, like the present, is regarded by some as a time of moral decline. Such paralleling is a tempting exercise but cannot be carried satisfactorily to any useful length. No indices of promiscuity such as those used today – illegitimacy and venereal disease figures – are available for the Restoration. Impressions abound, but these can be notoriously misleading. Kinsey[59] found little difference in sex behaviour between one generation and the next. This is hardly surprising. It is a historical truism that social changes occur but gradually, and always overlap, one period with another. Attitudes, and no less conduct, vary too between the classes, and the content of these is subject to change. The middle classes for instance have grown numerically, proportionately and in social influence.

Such phrases for venereal disease as 'loathsome' and 'filthy' were typical of the earlier part of the seventeenth century. In the eighteenth, however, greater tolerance prevailed. Indeed, there was an easy-going, light-hearted, satirical and even frivolous approach to sex and infection. This is clearly reported, for example, in Boswell's *London Diary*. Morals were generally considered lax, although this may well be – as some might argue of the present time – more evident in the literature and writing than in the actions of the people.

In the nineteenth century V.D. was again sinful and degrading and to be kept secret at all costs. Indeed the word 'venereal' was unprintable. There was a tendency to emphasize – some think, over-emphasize – the consequences of the diseases. In company with this general attitude of sexual intolerance was a moral bias against the female. For a man venereal disease was, at the least, a tragedy; at the most, a sign of depravity. For a woman it was a crime. Indeed it was widespread practice to punish 'disorderly and profligate women' by making them wear yellow dresses. Thus the requisite female wards of the workhouses were called the 'canary wards'.[30]

Victorian moral stricture was followed by the harshness of the law. Prompted by the excessively high rates of infection in soldiers and sailors, the Government of the day passed the Contagious Diseases Act in 1864, an Act 'for the prevention of contagious disease'. This coy subtitle, it was explained later, meant 'venereal disease, including gonorrhoea'. The Act concerned itself with certain naval and military stations. It provided for the arrest of women suspected of spreading infection, their compulsory examination before the justices and their detention in certain hospitals. Many people were incensed.

Those with reforming zeal in the liberal movements of the time reacted powerfully. Mrs Josephine Butler (1828–1906), who formed the Ladies' National Association in 1869, headed the 'Abolitionists'. She claimed that defenceless and under-privileged citizens were being deprived of their constitutional rights of freedom of action. A Royal Commission was set up in 1870 and sat for a year. Later a Select Committee of the House of Commons considered the subject of the agitation set in motion by Josephine Butler's pressure-group for the repeal of the Act. Success came to her in 1883, at a time when the services' infection rate was running at 27,500 per 100,000 men per annum. The Act was suspended. It was finally repealed in 1886. By the end of the century the services' V.D. rate was 9,300 per 100,000.

The Victorian effort to legalize segregation and isolation was a serious attempt at control. It was primarily designed for the protection of soldiers and sailors in garrison towns. Similar compulsory powers existed elsewhere at the time in Europe, and still do in various parts of the world, but in modified form only.

The communal conscience in this country was more fully awakened to the problem of venereal diseases by recognition of many medical disasters and no less by the high cost of caring for the infected during the First World War. With the presence of these factors, better understanding of diagnosis and the availability of new drugs, the approach changed from one of regulation and detention to the more liberal one of free advice and treatment. After sitting for three years a Royal Commission reported in 1916. Legislation followed rapidly on its startling revelations. Local Authorities were empowered by the Venereal Disease Regulations (1916) to establish free and confidential treatment centres. Financial help was given by the Exchequer. The principle of free access, that is, without an introductory letter from a general practitioner, was also established. Attendance of patients was to be voluntary. There has been only one period of exception to this rule. During, and for a few years after the Second World War, venereologists, usually through the public health departments, were able to arraign before the magistrates those named on two or more occasions as a source of infection who refused to attend for examination, and, if necessary, treatment. In 1944, for example, in England and Wales, 823 women and 4 men were notified as being named on two occasions. Four hundred and seventeen required to be served with notice compelling attendance. Of these, only 82 were finally prosecuted. The real worth of the regulation would appear therefore to be in the fact that it reinforced persuasion. In general, venereologists considered compulsory treatment as of little help in the control of the spread of infection, although Laird[63] claimed it useful in difficult cases. The British temperament is generally more amenable to sympathetic persuasion or at most social pressure, such as repeated visits by a health visitor.

Widespread acceptance of diphtheria and poliomyelitis immunization of infants is a prime example of successful persuasion.

With varying success and enthusiasm Local Authority clinics served the British public between the wars. With the coming of the National Health Service in July 1948 venereal disease or special clinics came under control of Regional Hospital Boards or Boards of Governors of teaching hospitals, as did many other Local Authority clinics and hospitals. Venereology was then established as a separate speciality. Thus from a beginning of 113 new establishments in 1917, there is now a comprehensive network of services of some 230 clinics in the United Kingdom.

To end this chapter on a note of realism will be a suitable prelude to examining the present position.

Few estimates are available as to the cost of venereal diseases. The U.S. Public Health Service [87] considered the cost of maintenance of the syphilitic blind to be 6 million dollars per annum and hospitalization of the syphilitic insane no less than 49 million dollars. This works out at about £18 million for the U.S. population of about 180 million.

In England and Wales in 1962 there were 138,210 new patients attending special clinics. The total number of out-patient visits was 791,000. According to Ministry of Health costing statements, costing depends on the type of hospital concerned. If all visits had been made to London teaching hospitals, the cost would have been £1·13 million. If all the visits had been made to non-teaching hospitals, the cost would have been £830,000. Thus without too much error we can say that day-to-day venereal disease out-patient services cost £1 million per annum. To this must be added in-patient costs, both short- and long-term. If these approach the American figure of £1 million per 10 million population, they must amount to £4·7 million. The estimated total of £5·7 million is for the year 1962 and for that part of the Health Service in England and Wales only. The loss to the nation in output and taxes, from those crippled and unable to contribute, and the loss to industry implicit in the 791,000 out-patient attendances, is anybody's estimate.

3   Venereal Diseases Today

Equipped with definitions and historical perspective, we can now consider the frequency of the diseases and their place and import at the present time.

Gonorrhoea is found the world over. Totals of new cases from many countries are collected by the World Health Organization and published at regular intervals. The figures, however, cannot be compared, one country with another, because the arrangements for treatment, and such factors as the provisions for the notification of venereal diseases, vary considerably throughout the world. It is possible none the less to study the trend in individual countries. Almost all reveal a high incidence of gonorrhoea immediately after the Second World War. Thereafter there is a fall which levels off about 1951–2 and these low levels continue for some three to five years and are followed, in many countries, by another rise. By 1960 the World Health Organization[117] reported such rises in fifteen of twenty-two countries. Three years later[118] it reported that 53 (47·7 per cent) of 111 countries and areas studied were showing persistent rises since 1957. In the same three-year period the rate had more than doubled in the Americas.

In the United States of America for the fiscal year 1962 the U.S. Public Health Service reported 263,408 new cases. This is 142·8 infections per 100,000 population, and a new high level (see Table 1). Seventeen out of twenty European countries (85 per cent) showed a worsening position in the same period. The highest and lowest rates found in Europe in 1960 were in

Sweden with 325·6 infections per 100,000 adults (over 15 years
of age) and Portugal with 9·4 per 100,000 total population. In
October 1963 a warning that gonorrhoea had 'reached almost
epidemic proportions in Europe', with 300,000–400,000 reported infections annually, was issued by the European office of
the World Health Organization in Copenhagen. Coupling these

Table 1 – Reported new cases of gonorrhoea in both sexes by year

	1958	1959	1960	1961	1962	1963
Germany (Demo-cratic Republic with E. Berlin)	28,167	26,973	25,736	24,893	22,618	22,085
Austria	3,709	3,635	3,923	3,994	(a)3,540	3,185
Denmark	7,291	8,194	9,055	9,244	(a)8,500	7,768
Finland	4,474	5,190	5,402	6,551	(a)5,702	6,458
France	(a)14,611	13,848	15,164	13,509	13,563	12,444
Iceland	144	98	189	240	(b)	(b)
Italy (c/d)	1,112	1,384	1,500	4,195	(a)7,027	(b)
Norway	1,910	2,137	2,173	2,714	3,317	3,160
Portugal	524	576	607	725	631	(b)
United Kingdom (c)	27,887	31,344	33,770	37,107	35,438	36,049
Scotland (c)	3,324	3,382	2,937	2,959	3,130	3,106
Sweden	13,038	15,421	18,510	19,662	21,474	21,540
Yugoslavia	(b)	15,847	(b)	15,958	16,722	(b)
Canada	15,040	14,826	15,661	16,460	17,697	19,411
U.S.A.	232,513	240,158	258,933	264,158	263,708	278,289
Japan	24,367	9,970	8,736	6,364	5,142	4,160
Poland	(b)	23,408	24,974	27,829	39,871	(b)

Some examples provided by Division of Health Statistics of the W.H.O.
(a) Provisional data. (b) Data not yet available. (c) Cases treated in V.D.
treatment centres only. (d) Cases notified in some circumstances only.

figures with a ratio of ten cases of gonorrhoea to one of syphilis,
the W.H.O. reported that 'the rising tide of venereal diseases
has now become one of Europe's most urgent health problems'.
    Increases were least in Africa, but parts of that continent have
long had some of the highest rates in the world. The Lagos
Federal Territory, for example, reported 4,907·6 infections per
100,000 adults in 1960.

There are exceptions to the general tendency to greater prevalence. A Polish report[14] of 1961, while stating that cases of gonorrhoea were decreasing, called for caution regarding future forecasts. As Table 1 shows, the fears were justified. From Bulgaria, also in 1961, we have a report[4] of a steady and continuous fall since the post-war peak to a rate of 29 per 100,000 in 1959. Available reports and statistics from the U.S.S.R.[119] give some idea of what has been happening there and how the problem has been tackled. The fall in gonorrhoea has not been spectacular but the incidence has been persistently declining from 81·6 cases per 100,000 in 1950 to 57·2 per 100,000 in 1960. Routine testing of women for gonorrhoea is often carried out in conjunction with tests for cancer of the cervix (or neck of the womb). In 1960 over $3\frac{1}{2}$ million people were examined for gonorrhoea in the Ukraine. The disease was found in 80 per 100,000.

A high degree of under-reporting must be expected from underdeveloped countries, with great disparity in the facilities they have for diagnosis, treatment and documentation. This does not appear to apply to Iron Curtain countries, where services, by all accounts, are uniformly spread and comprehensive. None the less, viewed globally, we find something of a general paradox, in that the more highly developed countries, with the best arrangements, seem to have the highest incidences.

On the whole the data available are held to be minimal. They give a conservative world estimate of 60–65 million infections annually.

Without becoming deeply involved, at this early stage, in considerations of the causes of present-day rises in gonorrhoea rates it can be said that developing awareness of the present state of affairs arises in two ways. There are those who investigate the problem in their own country, point out the medical and social accompaniments and pinpoint those factors which they consider causal. Other investigators consider these observations and seek the presence or absence of similar information in their own and other countries. Thus data are available on many aspects and provide lively topics for discussion at international conferences.

Briefly, the main social causes for the increase in gonorrhoea are to be found in increased and more widespread sexual activity among young people, especially, it appears, girls. A second and more obvious factor is immigration. This particularly concerns young, fit, energetic, unattached males. Both of these factors have been recognized as operating in Europe, albeit in different proportions in different areas. In Sweden and Denmark, with no immigration, the first factor is predominant. In England and Wales both factors play a part, particularly the second. Homosexuals also play an increasing role. There are of course many infected people who do not fall readily into any recognizable social category. These factors and the medical problems of re-infection and failure to respond to treatment will be fully dealt with later.

In England and Wales in pre-war years, the annual incidence of gonorrhoea in both sexes remained remarkably constant. From 1939 until 1945 the male contribution refers to civilians only and takes no account of the numerous infections in the servicemen of many nationalities then stationed in the United Kingdom. Something of the real prevalence of infection in the country during war-time is reflected in the steady increase in the number of females treated during 1941–5 and in the unusual 2 : 1 or lower ratio of males to females prevailing at that time (see Graph 1).

A study of reports from various countries shows male to female ratios varying from 6 : 1 to 2 : 1. These ratios usually reflect the variability, extent and standards of facilities as well as diagnostic and reporting methods. Not least is underlined the most important single fact about gonorrhoea: most females infected are asymptomatic carriers. Their attendance for diagnosis and treatment has to be sought, and this requires highly developed services. Ratios are therefore at their best where facilities are most adequate. Ratios have tended to come nearer to unity in England and Wales in recent years.

As Graph 1 shows, the post-war peak incidence occurred in 1945 for women and 1946 for men, and coincided with demobilization. As in other countries, the rate fell steadily to reach nearly half the pre-war average in the quinquennium

1952–6. The all-time low level of 13,964 male cases and 3,574 female cases was reported in 1954. From that year, with the exception of 1962, the curve of incidence for males has risen steadily year by year to levels above those of pre-war. In 1963 there was a higher than pre-war level for females. Present-day figures give a rate of about 75 infections per 100,000 of the *total*

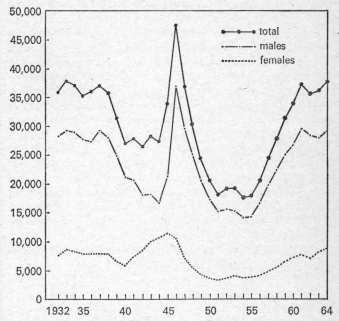

Graph 1. Cases of gonorrhoea dealt with for the first time in treatment clinics of England and Wales

population in England and Wales. This is a minimal estimate. A study of the year 1962[9] surveyed the work of 178 clinics in 145 large towns and cities in England and Wales and in Scotland. These clinics were estimated to cover 25 million of the population and the survey concerned itself with 90 per cent of the total reported gonorrhoea. The rate per 100,000 averaged 140 with extremes of 400 for the central London area and 50 for towns of 50,000 population or less.

Looked at from the epidemiological standpoint, we can say then that gonorrhoea is an endemic infection subject at times to epidemic-like increases. Exactly what constitutes an epidemic of gonorrhoea has never been defined.

Another way to view gonorrhoea, and gain some degree of perspective, is to place the incidence figures alongside those of other infectious diseases. This is not done in Ministry reports or in infectious disease reports in journals. The accompanying table (Table 2) is therefore a composite one. From the fourth-commonest infection reported in 1960 by the Minister, gonorrhoea moved up to second place, after measles, in 1961 and has remained there since. If present trends continue and hopes of successful immunization against measles are realized, gonorrhoea will probably become the most commonly reported infection in this country.

In summary, gonorrhoea rates in Europe range from 100–500 per 100,000 adult population (persons over 15 years of age). In several countries in south-east Asia, Eastern Mediterranean and West Pacific regions they exceed 1,000 per 100,000. Very high rates are recorded in some countries of Africa and the Americas. In England and Wales the rate for females is around 40 per 100,000, and for males around 120 per 100,000 of the total population.

What is the position regarding syphilis? Dr Guthe, head of the World Health Organization section for venereal disease, believed[39] that there were 20 million syphilitics in the world in 1945. This he based on reports analysed by W.H.O. and believed to give minimal data. The limitations of statistics on venereal diseases have already been mentioned. In the case of syphilis, this consideration is more telling, for the disease lasts many years. Perhaps the best index of its occurrence in any country is the percentage of pregnant women found to have positive blood tests for the disease. W.H.O. has sponsored numerous surveys of this aspect. The findings vary widely. In Pakistan we find 1·2 per

Table 2 – Notification of infectious diseases in England and Wales

	1960	1961	1962	1963	1964
Population	45·755 m.	46·166 m.	46·669 m.	47·023 m.	47·401 m.
		(thousands)			
Diphtheria	49	51	16	33	20
Scarlet Fever	32,166	19,984	15,303	17,437	20,172
Measles	159,315	763,465	184,757	601,111	306,721
Whooping Cough	58,030	24,469	8,347	34,736	31,597
Meningococcal Infections	630	651	575	606	505
Encephalitis	260	276	232	290	257
Poliomyelitis (paralytic and non-paralytic)	378	874	270	51	37
Typhoid Fevers	328	344	245	582	349
Dysentery	43,268	20,412	30,889	31,731	20,198
Food Poisoning	7,732	7,833	5,150	5,856	5,402
Gonorrhoea	33,770	37,107	35,438	36,049	37,665
Syphilis (infectious)	994	1,199	1,224	1,390	1,738
Tuberculosis (respiratory and non-respiratory)	23,605	21,747	20,519	18,937	17,599
Non-gonococcal Urethritis (males only)	22,004	24,472	24,494	25,289	27,166
Ophthalmia Neonatorum	1,063	932	1,017	970	832

Compiled from *On the State of the Public Health*, the Annual Report of the Chief Medical Officer of the Ministry of Health for the year 1964, H.M.S.O., pp. 32 and 210.

cent 'positives': in Hong Kong 2 per cent: in Burma 5 per cent: in India 2–15 per cent in different areas: in Morocco 14–30 per cent: in Egypt 7–15 per cent: and in Ethiopia 30–60 per cent.

In England and Wales in the post-war era the rate of positives was considered high. Macfarlane[70] working in the north-east of England found 515 (0·72 per cent) of 711,645 ante-natal blood tests to be positive during the years 1944–9. In 1952 his figures were 45 (0·28 per cent) of 15,812 tests. The Chief Medical Officer's report for 1962[88] referring to selected areas shows a steady fall in the last decade to 0·11 per cent positives in 61,872 women pregnant for the first time and 0·19 per cent positives in 48,433, women pregnant on a second or subsequent occasion. Although multiparae have always had a higher incidence of syphilis, only one of six cities listed in the report carried out tests more often in these women than in first pregnancies.

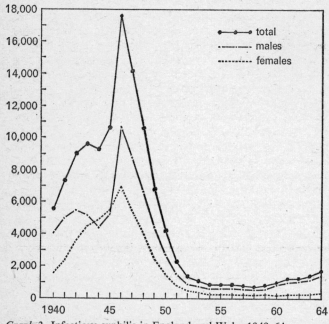

Graph 2. Infectious syphilis in England and Wales 1940–64

With the exception of Africa, syphilis receded after the war. Graph 2 emphasizes the dramatic fall in early syphilis in England and Wales after the Second World War. Much the same situation pertained in other countries and is generally attributed to penicillin and the resettlement of societies. In 1960, however, recrudescences of early infectious syphilis in the U.S.A., Belgium, Denmark and Italy were reported as occurring in the previous few years. In the U.S. fiscal year ending 30 June 1962, of 124,188 syphilis cases reported for the first time, 20,084 were infectious. This last figure followed a steady annual rise from the 6,250 infectious cases reported for 1957. This means an increase of over 300 per cent in five years. In Sweden the incidence of early syphilis in 1962 was the highest since 1956. In Portugal a similar story is found. In France, from a rate of 2·7 infections per 100,000 of population in 1955, the level was 7·9 in 1961. The number of cases is not large but a 90 per cent increase over six years shows the trend, as elsewhere, to be unmistakable. Comparable rises are found in places as far apart as Canada and Australia. Indeed, by 1962 no fewer than 76 of 105 countries were reporting rises to W.H.O.

England and Wales was no exception. From a minimal incidence of 704 infectious cases reported in 1958, the level has risen steadily to 1,738 in 1964 (see Graph 2). This includes 357 patients whose infection was judged to have passed into its first year of latency. The total figure gives a morbidity rate of only 2·9 per 100,000. The rise has been much more marked in males than females. In this country, and more recently in America and Denmark, attention has been drawn to the part played by male homosexuals in these increases of early syphilis. Nearly one third (half in London) of infectious male syphilis occurs in homosexuals in this country. The disparity between male and female figures is increased further by imported syphilis in seamen. A proportion of such cases are already under treatment when first seen at a seaport clinic. The number of cases of females with early syphilis has not increased appreciably. Infectious syphilis then, while not at present a major problem, could, if gonorrhoea is anything of an indicator, become so. The comparatively low levels of infectious syphilis in this country and the relatively modest rise suggest some measure of control. Due credit must go to the maintenance of our services throughout the 1950s when others followed a less far-sighted policy.

To sum up, estimated maximum annual incidence rates of

early syphilis have, after a post-war fall, risen to approach levels of the post-war years in some places. In the European region the maximum rate between 1950–60 was in Yugoslavia with 53·6 infections for 100,000. By 1962 the rate in Greece had risen to 22 per 100,000. In England and Wales the rate of rise, and the rate itself, is one of the lowest at less than 3 per 100,000 of the population in 1964.

There are many reasons for the different epidemiological behaviour of gonorrhoea and syphilis infections. Among the more important are these: gonorrhoea is the more infectious and in addition it has a shorter incubation period. The statistical chances of spread are therefore greater. The longer incubation period of syphilis and the fact that it is considered more serious gives time for, and impetus to, the tracing of sex contacts and their diagnosis. Thus treatment of syphilis sex contacts is more common than in the case of gonorrhoea.

There is, too, a greater chance that antibiotics will be given for unrelated conditions, or for gonorrhoea, during the longer incubation and infectious periods of syphilis. Thus the disease will be more frequently prevented, aborted, or rendered non-infectious. In the world as a whole many more people are in some degree immune to syphilis; for example, the millions in tropical and sub-tropical areas known to be suffering from, or to have suffered, such syphilis-like but non-venereal diseases as yaws and pinta. Furthermore, gonorrhoea, especially in the female, is difficult to diagnose and, unlike syphilis, does not readily lend itself to case-finding surveys such as those mentioned in the pregnancy surveys conducted under W.H.O. auspices.

In all other forms of syphilis the tendency has been for the incidences to fall since about 1951 in England and Wales. This is the accumulated result of improving education and better and speedier medical management in the last few decades. In this country a near exception to this general downward trend has been latent syphilis. The number of cases reported annually fell to 2,563 in 1960. There was a marked rise in 1961 to 2,903 but in

1962 the number was 2,578. Returns give no information as to the country of origin of the parties to whom the diagnosis refers. Positive blood tests for syphilis are known to occur as a result of yaws – a treponemal disease usually of childhood and common in hot and humid climates.*

Table 3 – Deaths from infections in England and Wales

	1961	1962	1963	1964
Population	46·166 m.	46·669 m.	47·023 m.	47·401 m.
	(thousands)			
Diphtheria	10	2	2	–
Scarlet Fever	3	2	2	2
Measles	152	39	127	73
Whooping Cough	27	24	36	44
Meningococcal infections	130	138	146	98
Poliomyelitis (acute)	59	18	3	4
Typhoid Fever	2	7	5	3
Dysentery	34	28	35	17
Syphilis	900	822	820	791
Tuberculosis (all types)	3,334	3,088	2,960	2,484

Compiled from *On the State of the Public Health*, the Annual Report of the Chief Medical Officer of the Ministry of Health for the year 1964, H.M.S.O. p. 226.

Many Commonwealth immigrants, completely asymptomatic and non-infectious after yaws, give positive results when tested for syphilis. It is noteworthy that 1960 and 1961 were peak years for immigrations to the United Kingdom. Thus the diagnosis of yaws was made 597 times to 1961 and 566 times in 1962 in the special clinics of England and Wales. These figures, taken with the unexpected increase in the diagnosis of latent syphilis, underline the difficulty of distinguishing the two diseases, especially in those from the West Indies and West Africa. Even a carefully assessed social and sexual history from the patient together with detailed clinical examination and other investigations does not always make the true diagnosis clear. As the

* The term 'treponematoses' includes all diseases caused by a treponema. The term therefore includes venereal syphilis, yaws, pinta, bejel, and several other forms of treponemal disease occurring in several parts of the world.

Chief Medical Officer's report states, the final diagnosis in such patients 'seems to be a matter of local inclination'.

With the fall in the incidence of late syphilis goes the frequency of death from the disease. Infections rank low as causes of death, totalling less than 0·16 per cent. As a cause of death from infection, syphilis is second to tuberculosis. Syphilis is commoner as a cause of death than all the other common infections together (Table 3). Its mortality rate in 1964 was 16·7 per million total population.

Chancroid, the third legally recognized or defined venereal disease in this country, is still common in many sub-tropical areas of the world. It was given as the commonest form of venereal infection in the forces serving in the Korean War. In the temperate zone of the northern hemisphere, however, it is not at present common. The cases seen are usually reported from seaports, occurring in merchant seamen or in servicemen arriving from abroad. Some idea of the decline in the incidence of this condition can be gained from the Swedish figures of 3,000 cases in 1919 to an average of 10 cases per annum in recent years. Some measure of our world-wide maritime commitments, as compared with Sweden, can be had from recent figures for England and Wales. These were 356 cases in 1953 and 135 in 1964.

Cases of lymphogranuloma venereum, although widespread in the world, appear to be commoner in tropical and sub-tropical countries. There are, however, few reliable estimates. In England and Wales the incidence level has varied from 76 cases in 1953 to 79 in 1964. Speculations that the influx of West Indians would adversely affect the downward trend have been shown to have little foundation. Undoubtedly immigrants have imported the disease but, like chancroid, many instances occur in sailors and are reported from our 'deep sea' ports.

While chancroid and lymphogranuloma venereum present little in the way of public health problems, this cannot be said of non-specific urethritis, a name sometimes contracted to N.S.U.

It is but one, but by far the commonest, form of non-gonococcal urethritis, or N.G.U., as it is called. Specific or identifiable causes of N.G.U. are inflammation spreading from an infected bladder, chemical irritation and trichomoniasis. It is, however, the non-specific urethritis cases which are largely responsible for the steadily increasing prevalence of the diagnosis 'non-gono-coccal urethritis'. Incidence is increasing in many parts of the

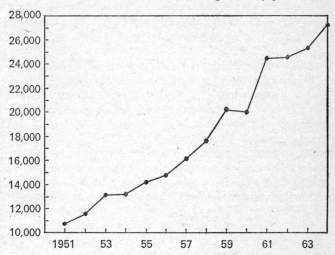

Graph 3. Non-gonococcal urethritis in England and Wales 1951–64

world, although official year-by-year national figures are almost unknown. In 1955 in a Far East study[32] it was found that N.G.U. was 3·6 times as common as gonorrhoea but this reverse ratio is probably not true for most other parts of the world at the present time. Hospitals and clinics in this country have made annual returns since 1952, notifying the number of cases of N.G.U. From a total of 10,794 cases occurring in 1951, the number has increased to 27,521 in 1964 (see Graph 3). (It must be remembered that these figures cover males only, as a comparable condition in the female is not distinguishable from some other causes of inflammation.) The corresponding figures for male gonorrhoea are 14,975 in 1951 and 29,050 in 1964. Whilst gonorrhoea is the more common disease in our big cities, N.G.U. is the more common in some county and county borough areas, that is, in those parts of the country where gonorrhoea appears to be more readily controlled.

There is no doubt that the Ministry figures give a minimal estimate of N.G.U. Some cases are believed to be asymptomatic and are found only on examination or when complications call for investigation of the genito-urinary organs.

Similar demographic difficulties arise in trying to estimate the incidence of trichomoniasis in the female population. As far back as 1947 Trussell in the U.S.A.[103] published the results of many years of patient study of the condition. He came to the conclusion that 'one out of every four or five women harboured the parasite'. This is higher than most estimates. Nearer home, an Exeter birth control clinic found 5·3 per cent of 562 women with the parasite. Other studies in London have given estimates of 12·8 per cent of gynaecological patients and 21·3 per cent of women attending a venereal disease clinic. American studies suggest that the condition is commoner in Negro women than in whites; in the pregnant than the non-pregnant; in prisoners than undergraduates. That the condition is world-wide there is no doubt. It is apparently very common in the more under-developed areas. For example, China and the Belgian Congo report female infestation rates of 30 per cent.

Of male trichomonal infestation there is less information. It seems that the parasite is unlikely to be present in more than 2 per cent of males. As a cause of non-gonococcal urethritis, findings vary widely from 5·5 per cent[79] to 41 per cent.[29] In seven series published between 1940 and 1959 and covering 3,500 cases of non-gonococcal urethritis the average was 13 per cent.[55]

Figures for incidence of trichomonal infestation are influenced to some extent by the methods of selection of the groups studied and, of course, by the methods of examination and how often these are carried out. At a most conservative estimate it can be held certain that over a million people in this country harbour the parasite at any one time.

About 230 so-called special clinics exist in the U.K. for the diagnosis and out-patient treatment of all forms of sexually transmitted disease. Terms like 'venereal disease' or 'V.D. clinic' or 'special treatment centre' have been generally abandoned. Such terminology as 'special clinic' is the most popular but in some places names such as 'Ward 45' or 'Lydia department', which are obviously much easier to use by embarrassed patients seeking direction, are preferred. In some large towns and cities facilities exist in 'diagnostic centres' for the care of patients by appointment. All such arrangements are directed at encouraging patients to attend as soon as symptoms or anxiety arise. The service reciprocates. In a work study carried out in one northern university city the average waiting time in its special clinics was only ten minutes.

Siting and accommodation of clinics is often poor. Like hospitals generally, special clinics have had very low priority in our re-building programme. A few clinics have been re-housed in converted hospital premises. Only one new and complete department has been built in the last twenty-five years.

The annual number of new *male* patients attending the 200 special clinics in England and Wales in recent years has been about 100,000. Only about 50 per cent have suffered from syphilis, chancroid, gonorrhoea or non-gonococcal urethritis. Another 25 per cent have suffered from some other condition found to require treatment. The remainder required no treatment by way of pills or potions.

Those patients in special clinics diagnosed as suffering from 'other conditions requiring treatment' are widely representative. Syphilis is a great imitator of many diseases, and this knowledge prompts many who have exposed themselves to consider the possibility of infection. Signs and symptoms referable to the sex organs also prompt many to attend for examination and advice. Genito-urinary and skin diseases especially fall into this group and a proportion of those require referral to other hospital departments. In recent years the increasing number of immigrants in large cities has put a great deal of pressure on the reserves of the V.D. (special clinic) services in those areas, as detailed examinations and investigations are frequently required to confirm or rule out the existence of tropical disease.

In the group reported to the Ministry as 'not requiring treatment' are many whose requirements are examinations, tests and reassurance. Many of these have simple and natural degrees of anxiety. Others are abnormally anxious and require much doctor-time on several occasions to carry them through to normal emotional equilibrium. Some require referral for psychiatric help. A small percentage of men in the group have been invited because they have been named as sex contacts of infected women. Some are the husbands of women found to have positive blood tests for syphilis at an ante-natal clinic. Others are the husbands of wives with trichomonal vaginitis.

The number of women attending special clinics annually in recent years has been around 40,000, of which only some 25 per cent have been found to suffer from gonorrhoea and syphilis. Nearly 50 per cent more required treatment of some other condition, the most frequent being trichomoniasis. As in men, the variety of conditions finally diagnosed is very large. The remaining 25 per cent of women attending, in whom no disease is found, do so because of anxiety or because they have been named as being in contact with a known case of infection and have been invited. The function of hospital clinics in excluding infection, by examination and tests, in those who have taken risks, and in reassuring anxious patients, is a major and important part of their work.

The total number of patients dealt with for the first time in any centre in England and Wales has been, therefore, around 140,000 per annum in the last few years. In a population of some 47 million this works out, allowing for re-infections and double infections, at about one person in 550 per annum. Nearly $\frac{3}{4}$ million out-patient attendances are made annually at special clinics.

The figures quoted for this country have all been obtained from official sources, but this is not the whole story. Figures obtained from hospital service clinics do not take into account those who seek care elsewhere, for example; in the services, at sea and from other doctors, both general and specialist, inside and outside the National Health Service. The Venereologists' Group of the British Medical Association in conjunction with the Medical Society for the Study of Venereal Diseases surveyed this aspect and reported in 1958.[102] The report showed that at that time there would be a rise of one quarter in the numbers for syphilis patients and one seventh in the numbers for gonorrhoea and non-gonococcal urethritis, if all other cases were added. The conclusion was 'The annual statistics of the Ministry of Health giving numbers of infections treated in clinics in England and Wales do not indicate the full incidence of venereal disease but seriously underestimate the problem, especially in the case of syphilis.' With the changing social circumstances since that report comes a recent request by the Ministry of Health for an up-to-date re-appraisal of this aspect.

In this chapter the main concern has been to take a wide look at the venereal and other sexually transmitted diseases and to learn something of their incidence patterns from a variety of sources. Emphasis has been laid on the recent past and especially on changes in this country. These facts will form the nucleus around which to build a comprehensive appreciation of what sex-transmission of disease means to the individual.

4 Principally about Gonorrhoea

In both males and females gonorrhoea is primarily an infection of the genito-urinary organs. If untreated, it may give rise to local, internal or more distant complications. Transmission of infection takes place from one person to another during sexual intercourse. Natural moisture or discharge, containing the living germs, is deposited, by the already infected person, on to the genitals of his or her sex partner during the act of coitus.

Rare modes of transmission are recognized. Parents or attendants suffering from the disease may, on occasion, transmit the germ by their hands while attending to girl children's toilet needs or when lying in close contact with them. Sufferers may rarely infect their own eyes or those of their babies manually. All these means of transmission are uncommon. Infection of adults by articles which have been in contact with infected persons and their discharges, such as clothing, lavatory seats and towels, is very rare, if indeed it happens at all.

The reason for the rarity of non-sexual transmission lies in the fact that the responsible organism, the gonococcus, is very delicate. When infectious discharge dries on a contaminated article, the gonococcus rapidly dies. It is likewise very susceptible to even small falls in the temperature of its surroundings, and rapidly dies when away from the body's warmth. It is readily killed by even weak antiseptics when they come in direct contact with it.

For an understanding of the infectious state and those complications localized in the genito-urinary organs, some knowledge of the anatomy and physiology of these organs and their

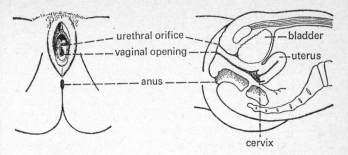

Figure 1. Genito-urinary organs in the human female

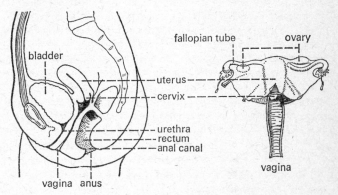

Figure 2. Genito-urinary organs in the human female

neighbouring structures is essential. Figures 1 and 2 show the external and internal arrangements in the female. The urethra is that short canal or tube of some 1 to $1\frac{1}{2}$ ins. (about 3 cm.) which extends from the neck of the bladder to the exterior. When a woman is standing erect the urethra runs downwards and forwards to open at the upper or front part of the vestibule of the vulva between the clitoris and the opening of the vagina. On each side of the external urinary orifice is the opening of a very small gland. In each cheek of the vulva there is a fairly substantial gland – a gland of Bartholin, so named after its discoverer.

These two glands of Bartholin each open by a small duct or channel at the side of the vaginal opening. The normal function of Bartholin's glands is to produce and supply a lubricant which makes penile penetration, and intercourse, easy and comfortable.

With the woman in the upright position, the vagina runs from the exterior in an upwards and slightly backwards direction, or, if one views it from 'inside', downwards and slightly forward parallel to the urethra. Its posterior wall of about $5\frac{1}{2}$ ins. (14 cm.) is half as long again as the anterior wall. These two walls are normally in apposition, but the vagina dilates easily, particularly in a backwards direction. The natural moisture or secretion of the adult vagina is slightly acid and an organism as fragile as the gonococcus cannot very readily live in it. Opening into the upper end of the anterior wall of the vagina is the cervix or neck of the uterus or womb. At the lower, free, end of the cervix is the opening of the cervical canal which leads through the cervix into the body of the uterus. This cervical canal is the commonest site of early acute uncomplicated gonorrhoea in a woman. It has an alkaline secretion, very favourable to the support of life and reproduction of the gonococcus.

The uterus, or womb, is a pear-shaped organ nearly as big as a clenched fist. It is fairly mobile but its natural tendency is to lean forward towards the bladder. It is suspended within the cavity formed by the pelvic bones by two broad ligaments running sideways. Included in each ligament is a tube leading from the body of the uterus to the abdomen or belly. These tubes are called the Fallopian tubes after the name of their discoverer. Inflammation of the tubes from any cause is called salpingitis. Behind each broad, suspending, ligament lies an oval-shaped ovary about 2 ins. (5 cm.) long. The ovaries are the storehouses of ova or eggs. In them each ovum, in turn, develops and matures. When ripe, usually some fourteen days before a menstrual period, an ovum or egg is 'laid', that is, it makes its way from the ovary down one or other of the Fallopian tubes to the hollow body of the uterus.

*

The sites for early uncomplicated female gonorrhoea are the urethra, giving rise to urethritis, and the cervical canal, giving rise to endocervicitis. In many cases both urethritis and endocervicitis coexist. The majority of women with such early uncomplicated forms of gonorrhoea have no symptoms. This is probably the most important and far-reaching fact about venereal diseases today. Hundreds of thousands of symptomless infected females, probably about one third of them prostitutes, form the great world-wide reservoir of infection.

The incubation period of an infection is the time from contact with the causative organism until it can be detected in the new victim. In gonorrhoea, incubation takes anything from two days to three weeks. In the great majority it is two to five days. This applies whether the woman remains symptomless or has reason to complain. Of those who complain, discomfort on passing water is not an unusual symptom. In others, vaginal discharge, amounting to more than is usually experienced at the height of normal fluctuations, may attract attention. For many a woman, however, the mild nature of the symptoms does not reach awareness unless she is advised by an infected man to seek medical attention.

Where an unsuspecting woman harbours the infection, or for some other reason goes untreated, several possible sites of local complications are available. The glands at the external opening of an inflamed urethra may become infected with formation of small abscesses. Discomfort or pain on urinating may be experienced. Inflammation of one or both Bartholin glands gives rise to one or two swellings. Fortunately Bartholinitis is usually unilateral. The gland swells to nearly the size of a golf ball and there is discomfort and pain on walking and sitting. Occasionally inflammation spreads up the short urethra, to affect the base of the bladder, and gives rise to the condition called cystitis, with increasing symptoms of urinary distress such as frequency of urination and burning. Rectal gonorrhoea may arise from spread of infected vaginal discharge or menstrual blood over the anus while the woman is asleep or defaecating. In such instances the secretions, containing live germs, seep into and along

the short anal canal into the rectum. Inflammation of the
rectum is called proctitis. It is not uncommon. Proctitis in
women is seldom a result of anal coitus, but some men and
women prefer this type of intercourse for reasons of variation of
pleasure or for the purpose of contraception. Jensen[49] working
in Copenhagen reported recently that he found gonococcal
proctitis in 63 (31 per cent) of 205 women with gonorrhoea. Of
the 63 women concerned, rectal infection only was found in
four. Ano-rectal infection, if it gives rise to symptoms at all,
causes slight anal discharge of slimy mucus or muccopus. The
discharge may be more noticeable in the stools. Anal irritation
and sometimes anal warts may be noted by the patient.

By far the most serious complication in a woman is an internal
one. It is inflammation of the Fallopian tubes or salpingitis. In
such cases the disease has spread from the cervical canal up
through the uterus without, apparently, doing much damage to
that organ. Not surprisingly, salpingitis has become common
with the rise in the incidence of gonorrhoea. As well as this
relative rise, there is, many believe, an absolute rise also. A 1960
W.H.O. publication[35] placed the current incidence of salpingitis
as high as 10 per cent of all cases of female gonorrhoea.

Salpingitis may be acute, subacute or chronic. In the acute
form it may be difficult to distinguish from other forms of acute
abdominal emergencies, such as acute appendicitis or ruptured
tubal pregnancy. The affected women, like so many with
gonorrhoea, may have had no prior symptoms before becoming
acutely ill with low abdominal pain on one or both sides,
perhaps vomiting, and fever. The subacute form of salpingitis
gives rise to repeated similar, but milder, attacks over several
weeks or months. As well as low abdominal discomfort or pain,
there is disturbed menstruation, periods being too often or too
seldom and the flow too much or too little. Often there is complaint of low backache and pain on intercourse. The protracted
nature of the internal septic condition renders the patient pale
and toxic. Accompanying anaemia is common and there is
added all the varied symptomatology of that condition. If untreated, subacute salpingitis smoulders on into a chronic state

in which the patient's Fallopian tubes become twisted by scar tissue. They are thus liable to become blocked and so impervious to the passage of ova. If there is scarring of both Fallopian tubes, the salpingitis may therefore result in complete sterility, i.e. the inability to conceive a child. This occurs in at least 20 per cent of all those developing bilateral salpingitis, in spite of what is generally considered adequate treatment.

The diagnosis of gonorrhoeal salpingitis, like all forms of the infection in women, is not possible by clinical examination alone. Laboratory tests, that is, bacteriological examinations, are the only possible means of making an accurate diagnosis. It is seldom easy. In the subacute, and more certainly in the chronic forms, it is frequently very difficult. This applies even if specimens are taken at operation. The details of diagnostic tests and the need for their repetition will be discussed later.

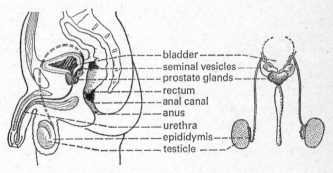

Figure 3. Genito-urinary organs in the human male

Figure 3 shows the relevant anatomy of the male. The urethra extends from the bladder to the exterior, a length of some 8 ins. (20·5 cm.). That part of the urethra within the prostate gland and for ½ in. (1·25 cm.) beyond is known as the posterior urethra. The remainder, mostly within the penis, is the anterior urethra. Many very small glands open off its length and two small glands stand guard at the external urinary orifice.

There is in each side of the scrotum (the skin-bag slung below the root of the penis) a testicle with its accompanying epididymis. In the body of each oval testicle, spermatozoa, sometimes mis-called male eggs, develop and mature in branching glands which unite to form some twenty small tubes. These join up behind the testicle to form a single thin-walled and finely coiled tube called the epididymis. This delicate structure is some twenty feet long and is concentrated at the lower pole of its parent testicle. In it, spermatozoa mature further. The tube now runs upwards from the scrotum through a canal in the groin into the pelvis. It runs round the wall of this cavity to the base of the bladder where it pierces the prostate gland. A branch of its terminal portion connects with a seminal vesicle, one of a pair of small sacs behind the prostate, which stores part of the semen. When a man ejaculates or 'discharges' at the climax of the sex act, his semen, some 2–8 millilitres, is made up of contributions from each testicle, each epididymis, both seminal vesicles and the prostate gland. Prostatic fluid only, which is sometimes required for examination, can be obtained on massage of the gland by a finger in the rectum.

The incubation period of gonorrhoea in men is no different from that in women, that is, usually two to five days, but may be as long as three weeks. With few exceptions, the man has symptoms. Usually the first thing he notices wrong is a burning sensation in the penis on passing water. Soon a continuous discharge of yellow pus from the urethra is noted. The man has anterior urethritis. Unchecked by treatment, the infection will spread upwards along the urethra, immediately under the fine lining, to the posterior urethra so that after a week or so of discharge and varying degrees of burning, urinary discomfort may increase to include frequency of micturition and even some degree of urgency.

It is fortunate that the disease in men usually directs their attention to the need for medical care, for there are many sites available for local, genito-urinary, complications. The glands at the external urinary meatus or orifice have already been mentioned. Many tiny glands open off the anterior urethra and one or more of these may be infected. Such inflammation may in-filtrate more deeply into the tissues surrounding the urethra. When such peri-urethral inflammation subsides the healing scars may cause narrowing or stricture of the urethra, a compli-cation common in days gone by but rarer today.

Infection of the posterior urethra is liable to lead to prostatitis, infection of the seminal vesicles, or cystitis. All these complica-tions are evidence of severe infection. Where the man has posterior urethritis the discharge not only tends to make its way into the bladder, but also into the ducts leading round the pelvic cavity to the epididymis of one or both sides. Epididymitis, as inflammation of an epididymis is called, is characterized by a hard, tender, red swelling nearly as large as a cricket ball in the scrotum. The swelling is heavy and painful. This is the most serious of complications, because when healing takes place, the scarring nips the finely coiled epididymis so that its correspond-ing testicle will almost certainly become non-contributory of spermatozoa. If both sides are affected, complete sterility is very likely. The parallels between epididymitis and salpingitis do not need to be laboured.

Chronic gonorrhoea in men is less common nowadays thanks to modern treatment and testing thereafter. Nevertheless some men do appear to have a mild type of infection only. At least it appears so, until infection spreads to result in the sudden appearance of epididymitis. Like so very many women, a few men may be dangerous chronic asymptomatic carriers of gonorrhoea.

Rectal gonorrhoea or gonococcal proctitis in men occurs almost exclusively in the so-called passive type of homosexuals, that is, those men who regularly or occasionally play the role of recipient or female in a homosexual partnership. Gonococcal proctitis in men is not uncommon. Usually there are no symp-toms and a chronic carrier state is liable to supervene. Many of the patients with this type of infection attend for medical care on the advice of an infected partner. The few men who have symptoms complain variously of slight anal 'wetness' or dis-charge, mucus and pus in their stools, anal irritation or anal

warts. Occasionally symptoms are acute. Not all passive homosexuals are exclusively so and proctitis and urethritis may occur
in one and the same patient. Catterall,[16] reviewing twenty-one
successive cases of gonococcal proctitis, found three with concomitant urethritis.

Complications common to both sexes were formerly all too
usual. They were not so in the early days of penicillin. They are,
however, being seen again with increasing frequency. In some
people gonococci reach the blood stream and eventually settle in
the joints, giving rise to acute or chronic arthritis. True gonococcal arthritis remains a rare if serious complication. It requires to be differentiated from other types of arthritis,
especially that associated with non-specific urethritis, to be
described later. Sometimes affected adults contaminate their
own eyes with their discharges and develop gonococcal conjunctivitis.

Gonorrhoea in babies affects their eyes. It is one form of
ophthalmia neonatorum, or inflammation of the eyes of the
newborn, defined by the Public Health (Ophthalmia neonatorum) Regulations of 1914 as 'a purulent discharge from the
eyes of an infant starting within twenty-one days of birth'. Less
than a third of such cases are due to gonococcal infection. The
mechanism is that small glands in the mother's cervical canal
are opened up when the canal is stretched to permit the birth of
the child. Infected material from these glands contaminates the
baby's eyes. In the earlier part of this century, gonococcal
ophthalmia was a common cause of childhood blindness.
Special care has long been taken to swab every baby's eyes
immediately it is born. If, in spite of this, infection occurs, the
eyesight can be saved by early diagnosis and modern therapy.

In girls before puberty, that is, before they begin to men-
struate, gonorrhoea takes the form of inflammation of the
vulva and the vagina. The child's complaint is usually of irritation, discomfort on passing water, or frank yellow vaginal discharge. The usual background story in such childhood infections
is that the girl has recently shared a bed or bath and towel with

an infected adult or sibling. In some instances there is a history of sexual assault.

Symptoms referable to the genito-urinary organs, and even clinical evidence of their infection together with a story of recent sexual intercourse, do not necessarily mean that gonorrhoea is present. Diagnosis, based solely on sex history, symptoms and signs, is always inadequate, often inaccurate and sometimes dangerous. In view of the epidemiological, social, marital and legal problems which may be associated with any single infection it is generally held as wise that every effort be made to secure a scientific diagnosis. Only adequate laboratory tests can ensure this. These are of three types. Microscopic examination of material, such as discharge or scrapings, from potentially infected organs is the most usual. Attempts at culture or growth of the organism in the laboratory from similar specimens is also regular practice. Blood tests for gonorrhoea may on occasion be employed. It is worth looking at the details of these diagnostic methods.

Gonorrhoea is essentially a disease of linings of genito-urinary organs. It spreads immediately under the surface of these linings and is called a sub-mucus infection. Material for examination, bacteriologically, therefore may be discharges of pus or scrapings from wall of urethra or rectum in men, and from the urethra, cervical canal and occasionally the rectum in women. Material is collected by a small sterile platinum wire loop or by a thin wooden probe dressed at one end with sterile cotton wool. Such material as is obtained is smeared on glass slides 1 × 3 ins. (2·54 × 7·6 cm.). When dry these smear preparations are stained by a standardized series of stains and examined microscopically. In early acute male gonorrhoea the gonococci are usually found without difficulty, lying both outside and inside the defensive white blood cells (see Figure 4). It is this material, together with dead and shed surface lining cells, which forms pus, matter or discharge. In chronic and long-standing infections, discharge of pus is less, and detecting the presence of gonococci may be a lengthy process, requiring repeated tests.

Examination of stained 'smears' is the basic method of diagnosing gonorrhoea. Correctness in the taking of smear specimens and their staining require experience. Examination of 'smears' is the only method of 'instant' diagnosis and opens the way to immediate treatment. Where specimens are poor, for example, if they are found to be contaminated, immediate re-examination and preparation of a fresh set of 'smears' for staining may be necessary. Finding the organism in stained specimens from females is not usually easy.

In a woman suspected of gonorrhoea one negative 'smear' examination is of very limited value. Gonorrhoea is a wickedly damaging disease in women. Any woman who has run the risk of infection, and who has thoughts and hopes of marriage and a family later in her life, will see the need for repeated examinations.

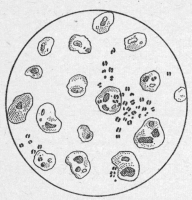

Figure 4. Pus from male with gonorrhoea. Diplococci (bean-shaped pairs) inside and outside defensive type white blood cells

The microscopic appearance of the stained gonococcus is characteristic (Figure 4). It is seen to occur in pairs. Each organism is bean- or kidney-shaped, the concave side of one facing the same aspect of its partner. Thus the gonococcus is commonly referred to as a diplococcus.

With the difficulty of finding gonococci in mind, one other method of detecting them is employed routinely by specialists. This method is known as 'culture'. This means that attempts are made, usually repeatedly, to grow the germ artificially in the laboratory. In the hands of experts this method may show the presence of gonococci, not apparent even on repeated smear examination.

There is another reason for preparing 'cultures'. Gonococci have to be differentiated from other organisms which resemble them in staining reaction, shape and arrangement. The gonococcus is only one of a family of diplococci. All but one of these so closely resemble any other member of the family that although most of them rarely inhabit the genital organs the need for detailed bacteriological investigations is clear in many cases. This is especially so in marital infections, where the ever-present possibility of the legal proceedings of divorce make these additional tests obligatory. Thus besides 'smear' preparations, material is taken by identical methods, and attempts made to grow the organism on a specialized and highly selective biochemical jelly-like medium kept at suitable temperature and atmospheric conditions. The fragile nature of the gonococcus makes it one of the most difficult of organisms to culture. The sterile medium in common use is based on a chocolate-like jelly mixture which is poured into shallow glass plates some 3 ins. (7·6 cm.) in diameter. The jelly 'sets' with cooling. These prepared plates can be stored in a refrigerator until shortly before use, when their temperature should be that of the room.

Specialized facilities for 'cultures' are not always immediately available. In recent years, to cover such a contingency, a special transport medium has been evolved. In it the gonococcus will stay alive, but not multiply, for as long as 48 or even 72 hours. Not only does this medium support the survival of the gonococcus but it depresses the growth of other organisms, such as contaminants which may also be present and which might otherwise overgrow and swamp the gonococcus. Suitably dressed swab sticks soaked in discharge from the patient can be placed in this transport medium in tiny screw-topped bottles which can be sent through the post. Like freshly taken specimens, the material on the swabs, on reaching the laboratory, can be spread freely on to the chocolate-jelly in the prepared dishes. These are then incubated at near body temperature and examined 24, 48 and 72 hours later. In the early stages the growing colonies of gonococci appear like dew-drops. Later they become more opaque and solid-looking. A colony can be picked off with a sterile platinum loop, smeared on a slide, fixed by heat, stained and examined microscopically just like a specimen taken directly from a patient.

Once grown in the laboratory, the gonococcus can be differentiated from all other members of its family of diplococci. Of four selected sugars the growing gonococcus will ferment only glucose. All the other members of the diplococcus group have different patterns of sugar fermentation. Culture and sugar fermentation identification form medico-legal proof of gonorrhoea.

The results of culture attempts are not usually available in less than forty-eight hours. Where transport medium has to be used, this period may be not less than four days. Recent attempts to overcome the difficulties of making a diagnosis of gonorrhoea at every patient's first attendance will be discussed later.

Blood tests for gonorrhoea do not have the same degree of diagnostic reliability as do such tests in syphilis. A positive blood test for gonorrhoea may simply mean that the patient has had gonorrhoea at sometime or that he may have it now. False positive results are not unknown. Negative blood tests for gonorrhoea do not exclude the possibility of infection. All in all, blood tests for gonorrhoea are very limited in their usefulness.

In all cases of gonorrhoea, and in those having repeated tests for the disease, the possibility of more than one sexually transmitted condition being present is constantly kept in mind. In women, for instance, other causes of vaginal discharge are commonly present. In men cured of gonorrhoea a urethritis from some other cause may remain. By the same token, all patients with gonorrhoea are examined for syphilis and are advised to have repeated blood tests for that disease, up to its outside incubation period of three months. Only in this way can the possibility of concomitantly acquired syphilis be excluded.

The aim of routine treatment of early uncomplicated gonorrhoea is a single injection of penicillin of such size and nature as to ensure the greatest percentage of cures in a large number of patients. In practice about 90 per cent of patients can be expected to be cured by an injection of 600,000 to 1,800,000 units of a moderately long-acting penicillin preparation, when this is given intra-muscularly. Larger doses are preferred in some clinics, especially for women in whom the duration and extent of the infection is less readily definable and who consequently respond less well to lower standard dosages. Some authorities prefer to give a large dosage on each of two consecutive days.

About 13 per cent of all varieties or strains of gonococci at present circulating in this country are in a penicillin sensitivity range which classifies them as being relatively resistant to that drug. Sometimes an area of the country will be specially troubled with a high percentage of 'difficult' strains, and in such circumstances an increasing number of patients will fail to respond to the currently employed routine dosage. Increased routine dosage in the area reasserts control. The general trend over the years is towards higher routine dosage in many parts of the world. In some places injections of penicillin are repeated over two or more days. In some patients initial response to treatment is followed after only a few days by relapse. No strain of gonococcus, however, has yet been found totally resistant to penicillin.

In spite of these recent drawbacks penicillin continues to be the drug of first choice for gonorrhoea in most parts of the world. It has one overwhelming advantage: treatment by injection eliminates all the dangers of misuse and carelessness or forgetfulness so readily associated with the taking of tablets.

Until a few years ago streptomycin was the second favourite. However, in the recent past it has been noted that nearly half the cases partially resistant to penicillin are completely resistant to streptomycin. Also the total number of strains resistant to streptomycin is increasing year by year absolutely. Streptomycin has the one great advantage of having no lethal effect on the organism of syphilis and it has a special place where there is a real fear, or suggestion of, a dual infection: there is in such instances the possibility of penicillin masking syphilis. Like other antibiotics, streptomycin is useful where the patient is allergic or sensitive to penicillin.

The tetracycline group of antibiotics is generally considered too painful for routine intra-muscular injection. These antibiotics, or others, can, however, be prescribed to be taken by mouth at six-hourly intervals. The problems here are twofold – the efficacy of the total dosage of the drug and the reliability of the patient. Patients may be forgetful about times; they may fall asleep; fail to set an alarm clock; be unable to take tablets without arousing suspicion among other members of their household or prematurely discontinue taking the tablets.

All drugs available are much more costly than penicillin. It certainly approaches the ideal. It rapidly renders the patient non-infectious. Its cure rate is high. It is available in a form suitable for injection. It is safe, and has few side effects.

From what has been said, it will be appreciated that the diagnosis of gonorrhoea can be made in many cases at the patient's first attendance at a specially equipped consulting-room in hospital or elsewhere, and that treatment can be effectively completed, in uncomplicated cases, on an out-patient basis. Complicated cases such as salpingitis or arthritis may require hospitalization and more prolonged treatment as well as general nursing and, sometimes, surgical care.

The absence of symptoms after treatment is no guarantee of cure. Repeated examinations and tests, by both 'smear' and 'culture' in the weeks after treatment, are essential to proper care. Only the fulfilment of such criteria can lead to confident assurance of a healthy future. This is especially important for the treated woman. If it is difficult to find the organism before treatment, it is by the same token difficult to declare bacteriological cure. The joint expertise of clinician and laboratory worker is essential. This problem and that of tracing and treating the sex contacts of the infected will be dealt with in detail later.

Chancroid, or soft sore, has a recognized organismal cause giving rise to genital ulceration and enlargement of local glands in one or both groins. The condition is usually incubated in two to five days. It is a disease so much commoner in men that one is forced to conclude that many women must be asymptomatic carriers.

The ulcer, usually on the penis, is characterized by rapid spread and enlargement. The ulcer edge is generally ragged and the base has a honeycombed appearance. Pain is a striking feature. This, together with rapid loss of tissue, generally means the man presents himself with the minimum of delay. In some, even where the sore is less acute, enlarged glands in the groin are found. If allowed to run their course, these glands become matted together and eventually discharge pus, if this is not removed by aspiration with a syringe and needle.

The diagnosis can usually be made on clinical grounds but a skin test is available in doubtful cases. Syphilis as a possible diagnosis must be excluded. Treatment presents little difficulty. Sulphonamides, streptomycin or one of the newer antibiotics already mentioned as occasionally employed in gonorrhoea are among the favourites. Treatment must extend over at least seven days if relapse is to be avoided. Follow-up with examinations and blood tests for syphilis are essential to completion of cure.

The relatively large virus of lymphogranuloma venereum belongs to a group which includes a virus affecting parrots and other birds, causing fever and pneumonia in humans. One member of this group of viruses causes trachoma, an eye disease which may be complicated by blindness.

Lymphogranuloma venereum is usually transmitted sexually, and appears firstly as an evanescent small lesion of the genitals usually after a week but in some a month or more. Enlargements

c

of the glands in one or both groins follows within a few weeks and there may be late suppuration or pus formation. In women, where the initial lesion is more often internal, the glands in the pelvis are more commonly involved. Untreated, such complications may eventually lead to deep scarring and narrowing of the rectum after many years. In the early stage the diagnosis can be made by clinical appearance together with a skin test and more certainly by a blood test. Occasionally it is possible to grow the virus from pus obtained from one of the patient's groin glands. Such pus is injected into specially incubated hens' eggs, for culture and subsequent identification purposes.

The two forms of drug therapy most usually employed are one of the tetracyclines or one of the sulphonamides. It is usual nowadays to give two courses of treatment, each of about ten days, with an interval of two weeks. This routine considerably reduces the chances of relapse. Again follow-up observation is essential.

5   Principally about Syphilis

A young man or woman when first acquainted with the fact that he or she is suffering from syphilis not infrequently says with some degree of questioning awe, 'That's the worst one, isn't it?' This succinct definition of the most vicious and deadly form of venereal disease is, even if incomplete, certainly accurate. In more general and scientific terms syphilis is, in its early stages, an acutely infectious disease invading every system of the body. After a year or at most five years of intermittent degrees of contagiousness it becomes completely symptomless. While no longer contagious it is, in this dormant or latent stage, potentially transmissible by a woman to her unborn child. The period of latency varies widely from one person to another, but is measured in years. If still untreated the disease will, however, re-declare itself eventually in a proportion of its victims. In this late stage it is a chronic, disabling and for many a deadly disease.

In its early stages syphilis can be cured. In the later stages its progress can be arrested and useful life prolonged, usually in comfort. Syphilis is capable in all its stages of imitating many diseases and it is for this reason that, especially in puzzling medical problems, a blood test for the disease is frequently in-included in the list of investigations.

The organism or germ which is the immediate initiator and perpetrator of the lengthy process is one of the genus spiro-chaetales. The members of this group of organisms are, as the name suggests, spiral or coil-shaped. Members of the sub-group, the treponemata with which we are here concerned, have been thought by some to be two-dimensional, rather than three-dimensional spirals.[98] The treponeme of syphilis (see Figure 5) is called the treponema pallidum from its pale white appearance when seen by dark-background microscopy, a special technique which shows highly refractile organisms very distinctly and in their natural, living state. The technique of dark-ground microscopy is essential for diagnosis because the treponemata do not show themselves readily and clearly by staining and the trans-illumination microscope techniques, so widely employed in bacteriology. Treponemata can be stained by silver compounds, however. More recently a dye contained in Parker 51 blue-black ink has proved useful for the same purpose, but such staining methods are not in general use.

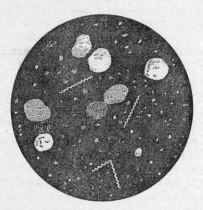

Figure 5. Specimen of blood serum oozing from primary syphilitic sore – showing treponema pallidum

A treponema pallidum, as found in syphilitic sores, has some-where between 6 and 24 coils, usually the lower range. The total length is between 6 and 18 microns or about the diameter of a red blood cell. The distance between the peak of the coils is around 0·25 microns and very regular. The living organism appears to corkscrew, alter length a little in concertina fashion, angle spasmodically, buckle and bend. In appearance and movement it is beautifully regular, sylph-like and graceful. Its size and movements are important in differentiating it from other members of the genus as a whole and other treponemata in particular. Several varieties of these are found in and around the genitals and mouth as normal or occasional inhabitants.

Unlike many organisms which afflict mankind, the treponema pallidum cannot be grown on biochemical media in the laboratory. Some animals, however, are susceptible to it. The rabbit, although liable to be a victim of a treponema peculiarly its own, is commonly used in laboratory studies and also for the purpose of diagnostic tests. In appearance the treponemes of syphilis cannot be differentiated microscopically from those causing other treponemal diseases, such as yaws, although the relevant organisms have individual names. Nor can the treponema pallidum be differentiated from those members of its sub-group, such as the Nichols variety, isolated in 1912 from the brain of a patient suffering from syphilis of the nervous system. This treponeme has been kept alive and thriving through many generations by being passed, by injection, from one rabbit to another for more than half a century. It is used in experimental and diagnostic work. Not surprisingly it remains virulent and is a constant hazard to laboratory workers. Another experimental treponeme, and a close relative, is the Reiter variety. This organism is said to have been first isolated in 1922 but its origin and its subsequent history is not clear. It is avirulent and can be grown on a relatively simple biochemical medium. It has been so maintained for years. Freeze-dried extracts of the Reiter organism are used in diagnostic blood tests for syphilis.

The life of the treponema pallidum is tenuously poised. It is very susceptible to drying, to heat above body temperature, to even mild antiseptics and no less to soap and water. All these destroy it rapidly. Moisture is essential to its survival. It flourishes therefore in such areas as the mouth, the genitals and the anal region. Syphilitic sores in these places are particularly infectious. The contacting surfaces of the sex partner of such victims are therefore very likely to be infected. Moisture is essential to the transmission of the living germ.

The reproduction of the treponeme is relatively simple. It divides into two new and independently viable treponemes every thirty hours or thereabouts. The two so formed become four, the four become eight, the eight sixteen, and so on. If at the initial infecting contact the new victim receives say 1,000 treponemes, by a further three weeks, when the first evidence of syphilis is likely to appear, the victim is already carrying a load of some 10 billion germs.

From what has been said, it will already be clear that infection may be inherited – so-called congenital or pre-natal syphilis. Much more common, however, is the acquired type of disease. The method of transmission in such instances is usually sexual. Accidental infection is rare. As suggested, the course of the acquired form is generally described as in four stages – primary, secondary, latent and late.

The primary stage usually begins some three weeks after exposure to infection. The treponemes effect access by penetrating microscopic abrasions of the skin. Marginal differences of a day or two may occur in the incubation period and depend largely on the state of infectiousness of the person initiating the new attack of disease and, no less, the degree of local skin damage at intercourse. Thus while an incubation period of three weeks is usual, a potential range of nine to ninety days is generally recognized. The primary stage is characterized by the appearance of an ulcer or sore. Since the infecting contact is usually sexual, the ulcer appears, in some 95 per cent of victims, on or in the genital organs. In about 25 per cent of infected women the ulcer or sore is on or in the neck or cervix of the womb, i.e., at the internal end of the vagina. In such instances the woman can have no idea that she has primary syphilis. A similar situation arises in the passive homosexual with a rectal infection.

The primary sore begins as an erosion which rapidly hardens and ulcerates as more and more defensive white blood corpuscles or cells pack themselves into the invasion area. So tightly packed are these white corpuscles that eventually they cut off the local blood supply and cause, by death of local tissue, the characteristic ulceration. The intensity of white cell reaction and the size of the ulcer varies from one patient to another but generally the appearance is one of a round, regularly edged, regularly based, often weeping, but sometimes crusted ulcer, varying in size from 0·5 to 1·5 cm. (less than $\frac{1}{4}$ inch to about $\frac{1}{2}$ inch). The sore is neither painful nor itchy. It is not usually tender to the touch. When taken between the finger and thumb the ulcer, and its immediately underlying tissues, feels hard and button-like – rather like a suspender button as felt through the thickness of an overlying skirt or trouser leg. Primary sores may be multiple and in some instances show an appearance much at variance with the usual. This is a vitally important fact. Most specialists tend to view every genital ulcer as syphilitic until it is proved innocent.

Primary sores, sometimes called chancres, may appear else-where than on the genitals. Homosexual men, playing the so-called passive or female role, may develop their primary lesion around the anus or actually inside on the wall of the rectum. Extra-genital primary sores may occur on the lips or within the mouth. Such sores are generally acquired by kissing someone with secondary syphilitic lesions in their mouth. Such people have been known to give dentists or throat surgeons accidental syphilis. Primary sores may appear anywhere on the body. Some years ago a man, twenty-two days out of prison, attended with a primary ulcer on his arm, near the shoulder, where his wife had given him a welcoming bite on the day of his release. In another case a baby developed a primary sore on the upper eyelid, being infected from a secondary skin rash around its mother's nipple.

In all cases the primary sore is of course a manifestation of the body's efforts to defend itself against the vigorously spread-ing and multiplying treponemes at their site of entry. Already at the time of appearance of the sore, many organisms will have breached these defences. Some may enter the bloodstream even at this early stage. The next line of defence lies in the local

lymph glands. When the primary sore is sited on the external
genitals or around the anus, the local glands concerned are those
in the groins. They enlarge one after the other, as multiplying
white cells muster in them, to try and kill off the advancing
horde of treponemes.

In the early primary stage all the blood tests for syphilis are
negative, that is, reactions are normal. Such tests do not give
positive evidence of the infection till it has been present for
some five or six weeks; that is, usually two to three weeks after
the appearance of the primary sore. To tell early primary
syphilis from other ulcerative conditions of the genitals it is
necessary to scrape all such lesions and examine microscopically the fluid or serum so obtained. If typical examples of
the living treponema pallidum are found, the diagnosis is clear.
Repeated tests of this nature may be required to establish or
eliminate completely the diagnosis of syphilis. The tests may be
negative if antiseptics or ointments have been applied to the
sore.

Similarly, enlarged glands in the groin may require to be
punctured and treponemes sought in the aspirated gland juice.
In some primary cases positive blood tests for syphilis will of
course be confirmatory evidence of infection.

Absence of pain or irritation and the slight or transient nature
of some primary sores may delude the patient as to the true
nature and seriousness of his condition, a delusion all too readily
embraced by some. In other cases the primary sore, untreated,
may take as long as three months to heal. Less than half of all
late syphilitics, however, have a scar bearing witness of their
original sore.

If undiagnosed and untreated in the primary stage, the disease
enters the secondary phase. Now the treponemes have broken
through all defences and are in every system and organ of the
body, multiplying at their usual rate. Clinical evidence of the
disease in the secondary stage is very variable. Headache,
malaise, pallor, loss of weight, aches in bones and joints and
low-grade fever may be experienced in one degree or another
and in varying combinations.

The treponemes, wherever they settle, are of course attacked by white cells. This is most evident in the skin where such individual little pathological processes form a rash. The type of rash varies greatly from one person to another and may even vary in the individual patient. Factors at work are the patient's reaction to the infection, the site of the rash, the type of skin, the state of personal hygiene and the duration of the disease. Syphilitic rashes tend to be distributed symmetrically. They have a typical coppery-red colour. A mother brought her 17-year-old daughter, saying that the girl had syphilis. When asked how she came to be so confident of the diagnosis, the mother explained that, apart from her daughter having the same type of skin as herself, the rash was on the front of both arms and not itchy. It was too, she pointed out, of the same brownish-red colour as the rash she herself had had at the same age. 'And that,' said she, 'was syphilis.'

Sometimes the secondary skin lesions grow luxuriantly in warm and moist areas of the body, for example on the vulva or scrotum. Such rashes, like those in the mouth, are amongst the most infectious of all lesions. Although syphilitic rashes are not itchy, in appearance they frequently imitate other skin conditions. Mis-diagnosis is therefore not unlikely. The mild and transient nature of some rashes may give a victim a false sense of security. Often concurrent with skin lesions are sores in the mouth and throat, sometimes with laryngitis and loss of voice. Enlarged lymph glands are frequently found not only in the groins but in the axillae, the neck and under the chin. In about 10 per cent of all those infected, other organs may be seriously involved. Infection of the scalp may lead to irregular, patchy baldness; involvement of eyes or bones may lead to obvious inflammation and pain; the blood-forming organs may be involved, with subsequent anaemia; hepatitis, or invasion of the liver, may lead to jaundice, and occasionally subacute degrees of meningitis may be present. Untreated, secondary syphilis tends to come and go with varying degrees of intensity and infectivity for up to four or five years.

Two methods are available for diagnostic purposes in the

secondary stage. Skin and oral lesions may be broken down by scraping. The blood which oozes is allowed to settle, and that golden yellow fluid part of the blood which remains on the surface when the red blood corpuscles separate and sink in clotting, is examined on a slide for microscopic evidence of treponema pallidum. Secondly, and as a confirmatory measure (it may take a week to obtain a result), the patient's blood is tested. Blood tests for syphilis are designed to determine whether the patient has developed antibodies characteristic of the disease. Such antibodies are part of the defences and assist in overcoming the infection by neutralizing its poisons and killing treponemes. Blood tests for syphilis are always positive, that is, show the presence of infection, in the secondary stage.

In both primary and secondary syphilis, great difficulty may be experienced in finding treponemes if local applications of ointment, especially one with antibiotic content, have been used. Similarly, oral or systemic antibiotic therapy given for any reason during the first few months of infection may, by killing off some of the surface, or generally circulating treponemes, mask the true diagnosis. In such cases, repeated microscopic examinations and blood tests for syphilis are essential as a means of determining whether or not the patient is infected.

Like other infectious skin diseases, the obvious manifestations of untreated secondary syphilis eventually heal. Unlike other infections, however, this is not the end of the story but rather the end of a chapter only. All that has happened in the case of syphilis is that host and parasite have reached a state of equilibrium. Attack and defence have resulted in an impasse; the flourishes of the early skirmishes are over and the real and protracted struggle is under way. Clinical examination at this – the latent stage – reveals no evidence of active disease, and often not even scars of the earlier stages; for primary and secondary lesions, unless suffering additional septic infection, usually heal without trace. Nor is there yet any hint of where treponemes are most actively engaged and where late complications may be expected. Investigative measures such as radiological examination of the heart and the great blood vessels near it and bio-chemical examinations of the cerebro-spinal fluid are normal. Only a repeat or confirmatory positive blood test result exists to establish the diagnosis of latency.

Such is the state commonly found in people who have had a blood test for syphilis as a matter of routine, for example, as expectant mothers and blood donors. Similarly a proportion of in-patients and out-patients under investigation are found to have latent disease.

Mr A. B. had been a blood donor for ten years and had given regularly. Routine testing of each donation had consistently given negative results. At the time of his referral he had just given his first donation for two years, and a routine blood test for syphilis had been found to be positive. Repeat testing of a fresh specimen gave similar results. Clinical examinations revealed no evidence of active disease. The history was non-contributory except for one facet. He had had 'piles' (varicose veins at anus) one year previously. These were probably masses of secondary skin lesions of syphilis. Mr A. B. was a homosexual. Eighteen months before, his musical interests had led him to spend two weeks at a musical festival. There he had a variety of sex contacts.

Mrs C. D. became pregnant for the first time at the age of 32 years. She had been happily married for three years. Her routine ante-natal blood tests for syphilis were positive. These results were confirmed on a second specimen. Examination revealed nothing to suggest con-genital or acquired syphilis and there was no evidence of late compli-cations of the disease. Her family history contributed nothing useful and her mother's and her husband's blood tests were negative. There was only one suggestion of possibly acquired infection in her medical history. When she had spent a year in South Africa in her early twenties, she had had a severe 'heat rash'. It was symmetrically distributed on the legs and arms, mild and non-itchy – really not a description suggestive of a 'heat rash'. She completed her description, influenced perhaps by hindsight, with a penetrating look that seemed to search for understanding and the remark – 'It was a very hot summer that year.'

Not all cases of latent syphilis are so readily diagnosed. Some times blood results to a variety of the routine tests seem to be in conflict. Some results are negative, some doubtful and others positive. Repeat testing is unhelpful. This type of problem may arise in congenital syphilitics who have reached adulthood untroubled by their infection, or, in latent syphilitics, whose natural defences appear to be mastering a long-standing acquired infection. It occurs also in people who have happened to have had penicillin in circumstances where some other condition has called for penicillin therapy. Their syphilis has been inadvertently and partially treated. They have had what the American specialists so picturesquely call 'happenstance' penicillin.

As has been stated, positive blood tests for syphilis indicate the presence of active body defences. At least three antibodies can be detected. Their function is to neutralize and finally establish supremacy over the infection. Healing of lesions is proof that such defences function well. Indeed, some patients seem to cure themselves with time, and many of their tests become completely negative. The course of the disease in any individual is, however, unpredictable and in so many the outcome is so disastrous that it is foolish to rely entirely on one's own defences.

The types of tests favoured by specialists vary in different parts of the world and even within any one country. The Wassermann test (W.R.) is by far the best known and the most popular. It is more complicated than the Kahn test, also a favourite. In this country, Price's Precipitation Reaction (P.P.R.) has replaced a wide variety of tests in vogue for instance in the U.S.A. The three tests so far mentioned form a group believed to be capable of detecting the same antibody. At least two of these tests are usually performed routinely on any single blood sample. The technical problems involved are centred around gaining a balance between the sensitivity of the individual test and its specificity, that is, its ability to detect syphilis without giving positive reactions in other diseases. These routine tests appear to detect a substance normally present in the blood but which increases to pathological levels in syphilis. The reason for doing more than one routine test therefore is to detect the nature and amount of the blood substance concerned. Two tests of varying degrees of sensitivity and specificity do this more ably than one.

In the last decade or two, great efforts have been made – as they have been made for half a century – to find a single test which would do this task rapidly, simply and economically. Perhaps the best of these is the test where freeze-dried extracts of cultured Reiter treponemes are used. This test is believed to detect a second and quite separate antibody. The Reiter test is certainly highly specific, i.e. it is seldom found to be positive in diseases other than syphilis; but it is not very sensitive – it can be negative in cases where the syphilitic process is not highly active. It can be and is used routinely in some places in conjunction with some of the already mentioned tests.

In 1949 Nelson and Mayer,[77] two American laboratory workers, described the Treponemal Immobilization Test. In this test Nichols treponemes are injected into the testes of a rabbit. After about ten days, during which the rabbit develops syphilitic orchitis, or inflammation of the testes, the animal is killed and the testes are harvested, as laboratory workers so delicately call it. The testes are shredded and placed in a vacuum flask with a highly complicated and delicately balanced nutrient fluid. An electrically operated mechanical device is used to shake the treponemes out of the shredded testes into the fluid. Portions of the highly infectious fluid, with its billions of living lively treponemes, are pipetted into small test tubes. To each tube is then added a small amount of a patient's blood serum. After incubation overnight, at body temperature, drops from each tube are examined microscopically. If the treponemes are immobilized, that is, believed dead, the patient is said to have an immobilizing antibody – a third and quite distinct antibody. The test in such circumstances is declared positive. The Treponemal Immobilization Test has proved invaluable in accurate diagnosis, especially in problem cases such as those giving conflicting results with routine tests. It is the most specific test available. Other conditions do not give false positive results. It is the one test by which the specificity of all other tests is measured.

It is not the type of routine test that every patient may demand but rather a court of appeal for laboratory workers and clinicians. The criteria for its performance are exacting and time-consuming. Every aspect of the pathologist's and the pathology technician's art and understanding is required for reliability. Even the most dedicated worker can hope to do no more than 100 such tests in a week – usually in two batches of fifty – for it takes nearly a day to prepare, a day to perform the readings, and half a day to clear up. The Treponemal Immobilization Test is generally called the 'T.P.I. test'.

The T.P.I. test remains positive for life in many syphilitics, and this applies to many in whom time and penicillin have effected cure.

Mr D. F., age 48 years, attended and was found to have gonorrhoea after a week-end in Paris with his bowling club. Of the routine blood tests, the W.R. was reported as weakly reactive or doubtful and the Reiter and Kahn tests were negative. Examination revealed no evidence of syphilis of any type or stage. He remembered using ointment prescribed for his wife's 'cold sores' when he had had similar sores on his penis fifteen years previously. He had visited his doctor shortly after this episode with a sore throat and enlarged neck glands. Penicillin lozenges were then prescribed.

Repeat blood tests gave reactions to Wassermann tests as before. The Kahn and Reiter tests results were again negative. The T.P.I. test was repeatedly positive. Mrs D. F. was found to have latent syphilis also. There were no children of the marriage. Mrs D. F. had had a miscarriage fourteen years previously, when more than seven months pregnant.

It would appear from Mr D. F.'s story that the true nature of his condition, while in its primary stage, had not suggested itself to him, or if it had, he had ignored it. The incident had not been reported to his doctor at the time of the sore throat, which was probably part of the picture of a mild secondary syphilis. Time and the penicillin lozenges had effected only partial cure. In Mr D. F.'s case the T.P.I. test was essential to the establishment of the true diagnosis.

*

From studies in Norway which will be dealt with shortly it is
known that in some 30 to 40 per cent of all untreated syphilitics,
the disease reappears in anything from five to fifty years from
its inception. In 1954 Dr Evan Thomas and his team working in
New York[101] made an attempt to determine the factors leading
to late diagnosis in 687 patients. Reasons were often multiple.
In 74 per cent there had been failure to find the cause in the
early stages. In some, the patient had failed to recognize his or
her condition or to seek advice when the truth was suspected. In
64 per cent there had been failure to hold the patient long
enough under care for early infection to complete adequate
treatment. Some patients had failed to cooperate; some had
been inadequately investigated; some had never been told the
diagnosis; others had not been warned of the finding of positive
routine tests. In 43 per cent failure of treatment was contribu-
tory. Clearly, responsibility for late tragedy appears to rest as
much with the patient as with the physician and the public
health authorities.

Late syphilis – the fourth stage – may be relatively benign.
This happens when it appears in skin, bones or subcutaneous
tissues. In these sites it appears as a syphilitic tumour which has
a predilection for ulceration. Such a tumour is called a gumma.
Injury may precipitate the appearance of gummata by upsetting
an otherwise happy symbiosis of organism and host. Gummata
have been known to occur anywhere in the body, frequently
masquerading as some other condition. Diagnosis depends on
appearance, blood testing and microscopic examination of a
piece of the tumour tissue or ulcer edge.

Coloured people, especially Negroes, seem particularly liable
to develop late syphilis of skin and bone as well as syphilis of the
heart and larger arteries.

While any body system may manifest late syphilis, the cardio-
vascular and nervous systems are by far the most commonly
invaded. Such involvement begins in the secondary stage. The
true incidence of late involvement of the cardio-vascular system
in untreated syphilis is not clearly defined. It is probably

between 10 and 15 per cent. If, however, every late syphilitic came to post-mortem examination, this figure would probably rise to nearer 50 per cent. One of the largest series to be reported in this country came from Newcastle upon Tyne. Macfarlane's team there studied 1,330 latent and late syphilitics. They were thoroughly and repeatedly examined and investigated by up-to-date techniques over some years.[71] Almost the same percentage were found to have non-syphilitic as were found to have syphilitic cardio-vascular disease. The figures were 16 per cent and 15 per cent respectively.

Syphilitic heart disease is more common in heavy manual workers. One cardiac patient in three or four also develops syphilis of the brain or spinal cord. While some two thirds of those who develop syphilis of the heart and great vessels do so within twenty years of first acquiring the disease, the onset of trouble in any individual may be as little as ten years or as great as forty.

The part of the cardio-vascular system principally affected is the aorta, that great artery which leads from the heart, curves like a walking-stick handle from front to back within the chest, and descends in front of the spinal column to the pelvis. From the aorta arise all the main arteries. The process of syphilitic aortitis, while often generalized, concentrates itself in the first part of the arch of the aorta. Normally this arch fills with blood, stretches and then recoils with every pumping stroke of the heart's largest chamber – the left ventricle. The wall of the normal aorta is well supplied with elastic fibres and it is these which suffer widespread destruction by the treponemes, to become replaced by more rigid scar tissue. Soon the aorta, under constant pressure, develops a localized, or a more generalized, dilated and baggy appearance. It becomes rather like an old and ill-used pair of braces or a mis-managed girdle in which the elastic tissue has been ruptured here and there by wear and over-stretching. The dilatations of the aorta are called aneurysms. Smaller ones may only be detectable radiologically; as indeed generalized aneurysms often are. The larger localized aneurysm sometimes obvious to the observer tends to erode neighbouring structure, both soft and bony, and not infrequently ends by rupturing.

Frequently the aortitis spreads to the heart valve which lies between the aorta and the left ventricle. This aortic valve, as it is called, normally closes under pressure of a blood-distended aorta, after each heart beat. Thus blood is normally prevented from leaking back into the heart's left ventricle. If the aortic valve is eaten away by the syphilitic process, it becomes quite incompetent. As fast as blood is pumped out of the heart, half of it leaks back, or regurgitates. Side by side with a worsening situation, the heart enlarges both in muscle power and capacity, so that more blood is pumped out per stroke and with greater force. In this way regurgitation is allowed for, or compensated. Eventually, however, after years of coping with this inefficient mechanical situation, the left ventricle fails and after several episodes of distressing threats to life, the patient succumbs to a state of complete heart failure.

In other patients, the aortitis involves the opening of the coronary arteries which supply blood to the heart muscle. These openings lie between the aortic valve and the commencement of the aorta proper. They are therefore specially vulnerable. The inflammatory process and its concurrent and consequent scarring causes constriction of the openings of the coronary arteries and diminishes the natural blood flow to the heart muscle. With the patient at rest no inconvenience arises, but when he exerts himself the blood supply required to maintain his more active heart in healthy activity is not forthcoming. Cramp-like pains, called angina, arise from the oxygen-starved heart muscle. Such pains may plague the patient for years every time he exerts himself. Syphilis is not the only cause of any one of the heart conditions described; especially is this so of aneurysm.

Cardio-vascular syphilis accounts for most of the deaths from the disease. Syphilitic aneurysms alone have been certified as accounting for some 500 deaths per annum in recent years. Happily, aneurysm is gradually becoming a rare condition, but not so rare that the new generation of physicians can ignore the example of the last who, ever mindful of 'the great imitator', ordered blood tests for syphilis as a matter of routine in all cases of heart disease.

If the cerebro-spinal fluid, that gin-clear liquid cushion which surrounds the brain and spinal cord, is examined as a routine in cases of secondary syphilis, about a quarter of all the fluids collected will be found to reflect the beginnings of an active syphilitic process in the nervous system. Characteristic changes in the cellular content and the biochemical constituents will make this clear. Untreated, at least half of those so affected will proceed insidiously to overt clinical neuro-syphilis in ten years or more. In so-called latent cases of syphilis the cerebro-spinal fluid may show evidence of as yet asymptomatic neuro-involvement.

Neuro-syphilis is a commoner complication in white than in coloured people and in men than in women. Some believe it to be common in sedentary workers – those who use brain rather than brawn. About one affected patient in five also has cardio-vascular disease.

Syphilis of the nervous system takes one of two principal forms. In the less common form the coverings of the brain and the blood vessels are predominantly involved. This leads to a wide variety of possible symptoms, from paralysis of a single ocular muscle to a paralysis of one half of the body. The commoner form of neuro-syphilis, however, is where the substance of the brain or spinal cord or both is directly affected. If this pathological process is concentrated in the spinal cord, it leads to a type of paralysis of the legs called tabes dorsalis. This declares itself in loss of coordination, due to interference with the nerves carrying deep sensations such as position of the legs in space, vibration sense and deep pressure sense. Balance is consequently difficult to maintain. At first the victim walks with a wide base, like a sailor just home from the sea. Eventually, however, he moves with a slow, wobbling goose-step as he tries to orientate himself in space and locate the ground with his feet. Sharp stabbing pains in the legs are a common accompaniment. Urinary difficulties and sexual impotence follow. The joints in the legs, deprived of their sensation, may melt painlessly, to become completely disorganized swellings, incapable of giving support. Tabes dorsalis is the commonest of all forms of neuro-syphilis. About 10 per cent of sufferers are also blinded by it. Since this form comes on ten or more years after the original disease, it is not surprising that it was many years before its true origin was known. It was from this form of neuro-syphilis that Adolf Hitler is reported to have suffered. Some would go further and declare his megalomania evidence of a more extensive neurological involvement – a combination of spinal and brain syphilis called taboparesis.

General paralysis of the insane (G.P.I.), general paresis, cerebral syphilis and syphilitic insanity are all names given to syphilis when it concentrates its effects on the brain substance. Here symptoms are, in the beginning, more obvious than signs. In most. they appear ten years or more after infection, either insidiously or, more rarely, with dramatic suddenness. In the majority, an initial period of headache, insomnia and forgetfulness is followed by faulty judgement and a lack of common sense. Where he was formally exacting about his work and dress, a man appears unconcernedly careless. In some patients the onset is an outburst of confusion and excitability, or aggressiveness and delusions. Lack of concentration is common and slurred speech often obvious. Some are euphoric, expansive and generous beyond their means or reality. Persistent delusions are not uncommon. Before long the whole mental power disintegrates. Mercifully the victim has no insight into his plight. Unalleviated by treatment, he slides into complete physical and mental break-down, to be delivered by pneumonia or some other infection from complete dementia. For those who have read Somerset Maugham's *The Moon and Sixpence*, this picture will not be unfamiliar.

Again the great variety of presenting symptoms in tabes dorsalis and syphilitic insanity casts syphilis in the role of imitator. Psychiatrists and neurologists need a high index of suspicion for the disease and routine blood tests in their departments are a commonplace.

The incidence of neuro-syphilis is fortunately falling today. Laird[65] reviewed the incidence of new cases in the Manchester Regional Hospital Board area during the decade 1951–60. He collected data from mental hospitals, psychiatric clinics, neurological departments and venereal diseases clinics. He attributed the slow and steady decline to the advent of penicillin and its employment in early syphilis since 1943.

As a cause of death neuro-syphilis is now rare. In 1964 only 27 deaths were reported as due to tabes dorsalis and 26 to general paralysis of the insane. This contrasts with figures of 120 for each as recently as 1955.

Congenital syphilis is transmitted to the foetus from the mother. The father has no direct part in the transmission. Infection passes to the unborn child through the placenta, that great fleshy mass which is adherent to the inner aspect of the pregnant womb and takes nutrition from the mother and transfers it through the umbilical cord to the child. The placenta is not fully formed until the sixteenth week of pregnancy and the child cannot therefore be infected with syphilis before that time. The mechanism is that showers of treponemes from one or other of the mother's organs are filtered by the placenta. In trapping them, the placenta itself becomes infected. Blood flow is interfered with and soon the protective filter-barrier mechanism of the placenta is breached. Through this gap in the child's main defence sally the treponemes to multiply and spread rapidly in the young and, to them, nutritious tissues. Overwhelmed by the invasion, the defenceless foetus succumbs. When dead, it is treated as any other foreign body. It is expelled. This is called aborting before the 20th week of pregnancy, and miscarrying when it occurs in the later months. Syphilis is of course only one of the causes of these conditions.

The more recent the mother's infection, the more likely is the foetus to be involved. In some circumstances the infection will come to it earlier and more severely. Thus in the case of a woman with secondary syphilis the foetus rarely escapes. In older infections the foetus may be infected late and even mildly, so that gestation could run its full term. In such instances the outcome could be a dead or diseased baby. Sometimes the child is born apparently healthy and it is not until it is days or weeks of age that it shows evidence of disease. Usually skin and mucus membranes are involved. If the linings of mouth and nose are affected, it is in a way very like that in acquired syphilis of the adult. The liver is also particularly vulnerable and jaundice may therefore be present.

Succeeding pregnancies in the same syphilitic woman tend to end more favourably, until in late latent syphilis the chances are at least 5:1 that, even without maternal treatment, the child will be born healthy. In the remainder of course, the outcome is so tragic – and no one knows which child will be affected – that all pregnant syphilitic women are advised to have treatment as early in pregnancy as possible.

Like secondary syphilis in the adult, the presentation of infantile congenital syphilis varies widely. It may be remarkably mild and pass unnoticed, so that it may be years, even decades, before congenital infection makes its presence known. An inflammatory eye condition, a similar deep affection of the ears and painful swelling of the bones are the usual methods. There may then be discovered other evidence of pre-natal infection. Characteristic stigmata may have resulted, for example, from severe involvement of mucus linings of throat and nose, with disturbed development of facial bones. The whole face may have the appearance of being pushed in. Scars may be detectable at the corners of the mouth and at the back of the eye. In some, the upper central incisor teeth develop badly.

Of the late, clinically active type of congenital syphilis, evidence too may be carried into adulthood. Scars of the surface of the eye may be obvious and may result in partial blindness. Deafness too may occur. Long bones, such as those of the shins, may be greatly thickened and bowed as a result of earlier inflammation.

Something of the misery of the syphilitic family is summed up in the medical student's *aide-mémoire* of the disease's complications:

There once was a man from Torbay,
Who thought that the syph. went away,
So now he has tabes,
And sabre-shinned babies,
And thinks he is Queen of the May.

(One can well understand that for the initiate some situations in life are too disturbingly tragic to be taken seriously.)

The outlook for the treated syphilitic today is excellent. For those who do not come forward or are not otherwise detected in the early stages the outlook may be disastrous. Recently an opportunity has been made to review patients known at the time of their early syphilis not to have had treatment at all or to have had only very small amounts of mercury and iodides.

From 1891 to 1910 a Dr Boeck cared for infectious syphilitics in Oslo. He believed that isolation, for the period of active signs, rather than the then available forms of treatment, was the right and proper way to deal with the infection. Thus he observed 2,181 patients with primary and secondary syphilis. In 1955 a Dr Gjestland[36] published an analysis of Boeck's work. He was able to locate the records of 1,978 patients. He followed up, in painstaking detail, 1,404 of them who were Oslo residents. Of 259 still alive, he managed to examine and investigate, personally, 216. For knowledge of the others he relied on hospital records, post-mortem reports and death certificates. He could define his final groupings as follows:

	Known	Partially known	Unknown
446 Males	72 Alive	43	72
	259 Dead		
958 Females	187 Alive	151	185
	435 Dead		

Of the total, 1,147 'known' or 'partially known', 15·8 per cent had developed some form of benign late syphilis, such as gumma or bone syphilis. Of the 331 men and 622 women classed as 'known', 9·2 per cent and 5·1 per cent respectively had evidence of neuro-syphilis. Of the patients over 15 years of age, at the time of their infections, 10·4 per cent had cardio-vascular complications.

Gjestland concluded that somewhere between 60 and 70 per cent of untreated syphilitics go through life 'with little or no inconvenience as a result of their disease'. This may be an over-estimate. The proportions of males to females in the series was 1:2. This ratio is the reverse, more or less, of the usual because more beds were available for female patients. It is well recognized that syphilis is a much more severe disease in men than in women.

Such excess mortality as Gjestland found amongst the syphilitics, over the population generally, he attributed to socio-economic factors rather than to the disease. Opinion on this point varies. American Public Health Service workers[96] suggest that the life expectancy of an individual of 25–50 years of age suffering from syphilis is reduced by his or her disease. A syphilis-free control group, matched for age and socio-economic background, was used in their study. Animal experiments purport to throw some light on the problem.[93] Under experimental conditions, syphilitic mice had a reduced life span as compared with matching controls. The experimenter believed that the reason for the difference lay in the part that syphilitic infection played as a general depressant of natural defence mechanisms. Thus the syphilitic mice were more liable to succumb to other infections.

To the question, 'What is the outlook for the syphilitic today?' the short answer is 'Never better'. In primary and secondary disease, modern therapy reaches near perfection with daily injections of penicillin for ten days. It is the drug of first choice. The cure rate with one course is put as high as 97 per cent, as shown by a two-year follow-up. Some specialists, aiming to cure 100 per cent in a short time, give more than one course. Follow-up blood tests are an essential to effect a cure, and these are usually carried out at monthly and, later, three-monthly intervals. Thus, initially positive results show reversal to normal negative and remain so. The cerebro-spinal fluid is checked at one year after treatment. Should a treated woman become pregnant before completing a two-year follow-up, it is customary to give her an insurance course of penicillin. For the peace of mind of all concerned, all babies of treated syphilitic women have a blood test for syphilis done routinely.

In the latent form of the disease, the effects of treatment may be remarkable, in a general way; the patient will rapidly feel and work better as his chronic infection is mastered. In the long and broad view, we can say with confidence that we will not now see hundreds and hundreds of late syphilitics as a result of last war infections, in the way that occurred after the First World War.

Those with benign forms of late syphilis respond very promptly to penicillin. Gummata usually heal completely in a few weeks. In the serious late processes of syphilis, treatment can be expected to effect arrest. Thus in cardio-vascular disease, angina may be relieved or the expansion of an aneurysm apparently brought to a stop. Here, as in the late neurologically stricken patients, much damage has often been done. Nervous system tissue is irreplaceable. None the less the patient and his relatives may look ahead with some degree of confidence. In G.P.I., for example, about a third of all patients are able to return to their original occupation and one third more can cope with some type of work. The remainder, sooner or later, become permanent inmates of mental hospitals. In late forms of syphilis, some degree of reversal from positive to negative blood test readings may be expected. Reversal of all tests to negative is not, however, seen as an essential criterion of cure. The aim of treatment in long-standing cases is to protect the individual patient from the ravages of complications. Residually positive blood results, often remaining so for life, are regarded simply as scars.

For all those treated for syphilis a minimum of two-year follow-up is essential. No matter how thorough the treatment and how well the patient has attended for it – most patients complete treatment on an out-patient basis – a small percentage always relapse. Some are re-infected. Early detection of these

states and their treatment will prevent any upsurge of infectiousness and safeguard the health of the patient and his or her family.
  When the patient is sensitive to penicillin a wide choice of
other antibiotics is available. All are regarded as second-
best. This is principally because they are generally available
for oral medication only. The element of unreliability, inherent
in such therapy, has already been mentioned when discussing
the treatment of gonorrhoea. Medicines ancillary to the
main antisyphilitic treatment are of course many. Bismuth and
potassium iodide are the only ones in occasional use nowadays.
They may be employed in selected patients by way of introductory treatment. Cortisone preparations are especially
valuable in preventing blindness in congenital eye disease. Such
drugs may prove useful in preventing deafness. Mechanical supports for disintegrating joints often slow down the process of disorganization. Cardiac surgery may be helpful in some patients.

  Allusion has already been made to other forms of treponemal
disease. Most of these are prevalent in other parts of the world.
Several have been and are being tackled on a mass treatment
scale by World Health Organization teams. These have been
very successful, as follow-up surveys show. The treponemal
disease of particular interest to us at present in this country is
yaws. It is a disease, usually of childhood, and passed by social
contact, rather than sexual contact. It is found among West
Indian and West African immigrants, generally in a latent and
sometimes in a treated form. Thus routine blood tests for
syphilis are reported positive in about 4 per cent of such people.
The problem of whether these results are due to childhood yaws,
or syphilis at some time, is not always easily determined. To
know the truth is especially vital in pregnant West Indian
women. Syphilis may infect an unborn child; yaws does not.
Where science fails to help us differentiate, reliance is on art.
This may resolve itself into making a diagnosis of yaws but
giving treatment as for syphilis. In this way healthy babies are
assured.

*

Positive blood tests, particularly positive Wassermann tests, do not always mean that syphilis is or has been present. A similar statement can be made about the Kahn test and rarely about Price's Precipitation Reaction. Such false positive results are sometimes due to technical errors and repeat testing on a fresh specimen will give negative findings. More often, temporary false positive results are due to some other illness. Almost any illness may cause them. At times they are found in those recently vaccinated or inoculated. Repeat testing shows the majority of these biological positive reactions to be short-lived and of no consequence. The false positive nature of such reactions is confirmed by repeatedly negative results to the more specific tests, such as the Reiter test or the Treponemal Immobilization Test.

More serious is the outlook for the *chronic* biological false positive reactor, that is, a person in whom the results of the Wassermann test, for example, are persistently and repeatedly positive for six months or more. Not a few such people give a history of vague recurrent attacks of fever, joint pains or swellings or skin lesions associated with rheumatism-like conditions. Investigation and prolonged observation are essential. About one third of such patients are said to develop rheumatism or collagen (connective tissue) disease later in life. Our present state of knowledge is such that we can offer chronic biological false positive reactors little more than the masterly inactivity of six-monthly or yearly observation with exhortation to care for themselves generally and more especially if they suffer from any infectious conditions.

6   Principally about Other Sexually Transmitted Diseases

Of the many conditions capable of being sexually transmitted, only gonorrhoea, syphilis and chancroid qualify for the title of venereal diseases. This qualification has legal standing. It stems from a recognition of the organisms concerned and the fact that their mode of spread is almost always through coitus. About the other sexually transmitted conditions, to which we now address ourselves, there is less scientific certainty. The organismal cause (or causes) in at least one is usually unknown. In another, the mode of spread, in some cases, is in question. Our present concern will be principally with these two conditions. They are non-gonococcal urethritis (N.G.U.) and trichomonal infestation. Several skin conditions capable of transfer from one person to another during coitus will be briefly considered.

It is probably near the truth to say that more than half, and perhaps three quarters, of all male cases of urethritis are gonococcal. Very few countries report their incidence of N.G.U. Ceylon showed a rise from 158 cases in 1953 to 784 in 1962–3. The rise paralleled that of gonorrhoea and formed some 30 per cent of the total male cases of urethritis. Since the figures for England and Wales are among the few available, they are worth quoting in full (see Table 4). The rise in the number of cases of N.G.U. has been persistent. Over the period shown the incidence of male gonorrhoea has approximately doubled, while N.G.U. has increased about 150 per cent.

There are several reasons for N.G.U. being more often recognized nowadays. Firstly, with the advent of penicillin, and the more prompt and certain cure of gonorrhoea, many cases formerly diagnosed on clinical grounds alone as gonococcal are not now so regarded. Secondly, N.G.U. is more often clearly and bacteriologically recognized as such at a patient's first attendance. Thirdly, there is, as well as these relative increases, an absolute increase in the incidence of the disease, at least in some parts of the world. Such rises have accompanied rises in gonorrhoea. This fact is quoted in support of the view that N.G.U. is usually a sexually transmitted disease.

Table 4 – Incidence of gonorrhoea and non-gonococcal urethritis in England and Wales. Males only

Year	Gonorrhoea	N.G.U.	Year	Gonorrhoea	N.G.U.
1951	14,975	10,794	1958	22,398	17,606
1952	15,510	11,552	1959	24,964	20,227
1953	15,242	13,157	1960	26,618	22,004
1954	13,962	13,279	1961	29,519	24,472
1955	14,079	14,269	1962	28,329	24,494
1956	16,377	14,825	1963	27,895	25,001
1957	19,620	16,066	1964	29,050	27,166

In the great majority of cases of N.G.U. no recognizable organismal cause is found. Indeed in only some 5 to 10 per cent is a cause detected by any of the available routine and standard laboratory methods at present available. Some 2 to 3 per cent are due to descending infection from higher up the urinary tract, particularly from cystitis, i.e. inflammation of the bladder, a condition which can be caused by a wide variety of bacteria. More common, however, is the urethritis associated with the protozoan trichomonas vaginalis which we shall discuss later. The remaining cases of N.G.U., with recognizable etiology, cover a wide range of which the following are the more notable – chemical irritation due to abnormal urinary constituents, such as sugar in diabetes, and uric acid in gout; antiseptics applied by the patient in a panic about possible venereal infection; foreign

bodies in the urethra; scars associated with previously complicated urethritis; intra-meatal warts and on occasion a primary
sore of syphilis. All these causes, and others, are rare.

Sometimes the anxious and introspective man produces a
'urethral discharge' by repeatedly squeezing the penis. This
traumatic process churns up cells shed from the lining of the
urethra. These, with adjacent natural moisture, give a greyish
secretion. Occasionally, in others, a sticky mucus may appear
at the external urinary orifice as a result of pressure by hard
faeces on the prostate gland. In yet others so-called discharge
may simply be an excess of normal secretion, associated, for
example, with whetted but unfulfilled sexual appetite. In neither
case need there necessarily be infection.

To the remaining 90 per cent or more of cases of N.G.U. –
that is, to those cases in which no discernible or specific cause is
detected – the name non-specific urethritis (N.S.U.) is generally
applied. The diagnosis of N.S.U. is made therefore by excluding
gonorrhoea, trichomonal infestation, cystitis and all the other
possible causes of urethritis.

Non-specific urethritis (N.S.U.) usually follows sexual intercourse by a period of incubation longer than is customary in
gonorrhoea. The period from intercourse to appearance of
urethral discharge may be anything from a few days to a few
weeks. In more than half it is over ten days. The relationship of
the condition to sexual intercourse is widely accepted. The
evidence in favour is mainly epidemiological. Mention has
already been made of the parallel rises of gonorrhoea and
N.G.U. in the last decade. It has been noted too that one man in
four or five with N.G.U. gives a history of gonorrhoea at some
time. This suggests an element of promiscuity. There are, however, reservations. In a series of 200 consecutive cases published
in 1958[5] some thirty-one of the married men denied extra-marital
intercourse during the previous three months. Fourteen men in
the whole series denied intercourse at any time during the
previous three months. The authors found no clear-cut correla-
tion between the sexual behaviour and habits of their patients
and the more familiar patterns of gonorrhoea sufferers. The

possibility of several different types or causes of N.S.U. arises from these and other observations. The mildness of the condition in some men may account for differences in diagnostic rates between one country and another or one area and another. Thus mild cases may be considered by one physician to be little more than normal secretion while another will label an identical discharge as N.S.U. It has been seriously suggested therefore that the diagnosis of N.S.U. may be, in some cases, one of inclination.

The list of suggested causes of N.S.U. is more than equalled by the number of suggested treatments – a combination in medicine which commonly accompanies poor understanding. Bacteria are always the first to be suspected as the cause of apparently infectious conditions. Those found in stained smear specimens of urethral discharge, however, are generally regarded as normal inhabitants or as contaminants of para-meatal skin or the first centimetre or so of the urethra. One group of bacteria has come in for special attention. They are the pleuro-pneumonia-like organisms (P.P.L.O), so called because they resemble those causing inflammation of the lung and its covering, the pleura, in sheep. These organisms have been found in varying percentages of groups of patients with N.S.U. Pleuro-pneumonia-like organisms have also been found in the urethra of a small percentage of youths presumed not to have had intercourse. It has been suggested that they become pathogenic only under certain conditions. In the female P.P.L.O. have been found in pelvic abscesses. Blood tests designed to detect antibodies to them have proved positive and have given support to the theory that at least a variety of P.P.L.O. plays a part in the causation of N.S.U. The case is, however, far from proven.

Another suggested theory is based on the idea that N.S.U. is a manifestation of sensitivity to some unknown fresh infection or condition, in much the same way that rheumatic fever may follow streptococcal throat infection, or urticaria ('nettle-rash') may follow ingestion of strawberries in some people. This theory has at present very little support.

Research to support a viral origin for N.S.U. has been singularly unsuccessful until recently. Sporadically, over the last fifty years, various workers have been identifying what they called inclusion bodies in stained specimens of cells obtained by scraping the urethra of males with non-specific urethral discharge. Inclusion bodies represent one stage in the life cycle of viruses. Repeated attempts by several investigators over many years to grow a virus from such urethral scrapings have not, however, met with any success. There has been a refreshingly new approach to this aspect of the problem recently.

One form of inflammation of the eyes of newly born babies is called inclusion conjunctivitis. For many years stained scrapings from such eyes have shown virus inclusions in cells. The suspected virus has been cultivated. It has been found to be similar in many respects to the virus of trachoma, an eye disease which may be complicated by blindness, in many sub-tropical areas of the world. The two viruses are, indeed, thought to produce a single disease whose appearance and progress is altered by climatic, nutritional, social and hygienic conditions. For these reasons the viruses are thought to belong to one family and have been called Tric viruses, 'Tr' standing for trachoma and 'ic' for inclusion conjunctivitis. The virus, or agent as it is sometimes called, is one of the largest to infect man. That inclusion conjunctivitis is acquired by a baby from its mother at birth is suggested by the finding of inclusions in scrapings of cells from the mother's birth canal. In some of the mothers the virus has been grown from these sites. Support is given to the sexual transmission theory by the finding of inclusions in, and occasional cultivation of viruses from, the urethral cells of the husbands of the mothers concerned. In some instances the men had N.S.U.[25] So far only a few families have been investigated by these techniques and the findings will need to be confirmed by independent workers. Further impetus and encouragement has been given to this work by a recent and substantial grant from the Medical Research Council.

Most clinicians who have given experienced thought to the

problem favour a viral theory of causation of N.S.U. Apart from what has been said, their views stem also from the response of the condition to broad spectrum antibiotics (a phenomenon common to 'large' virus diseases), evidence of latency, and the relapsing nature of the condition in a substantial proportion of the men affected.

Clinical examination shows that N.S.U. is usually confined to the anterior urethra. As has been suggested, the condition may be so mild and the discharge so little that it occurs only first thing in the morning before urination. In a few men the condition is asymptomatic. In others the urethral discharge is profuse and purulent and so closely resembles acute gonorrhoea as to be indistinguishable from it clinically. In yet others there is spread to the posterior urethra and, in a few, inflammation of the base of the bladder, with all the varied symptomatology of that condition. Epididymitis and urethral stricture from peri-urethral gland involvement are occasional complications. Some specialists consider that inflammation of the prostate gland is a common accompaniment of non-specific urethritis, either as a complication or as 'chronic from the first'.[58] To cover this clinical picture the term 'non-specific genital infection' has been coined. The diagnosis of prostatitis is made by examining, microscopically, a specimen of prostatic fluid obtained by digital massage of the gland *per rectum*. The number of white blood cells – so-called pus cells – found in the fluid is relevant. The percentage of men diagnosed as having prostatitis can be increased by examining five specimens obtained after a single massage. Those who follow these methods are not agreed on the number of pus cells required to make a diagnosis of prostatitis. In this country, however, advocates generally recommend, as the upper limit of normal 10-pus cells per microscope field, using a magnification around 1,300. Irrespective of their numbers, if pus cells occur in clumps this is diagnostic of prostatitis. The term 'pus cell' is perhaps not a good one. The cells found are white blood cells. Attempts to establish levels of normality in the number of white blood cells in prostatic fluid have not proved completely successful. In some reports substantial percentages of controls appear to have prostatitis. Oates[82] and Ambrose and Taylor[1] for example, when they used much the same criteria, found a third of their controls with prostatitis. Inflammatory changes in joint surfaces at the lower end of the spine are cited as evidence of spread of pre-existent prostatitis. It is postulated that infection spreads from the prostate gland by a network of veins.

There is a notable absence of reports claiming that treatment is beneficial in prostatitis. Ambrose and Taylor,[1] already mentioned, found that oxytetracycline therapy, while curing the urethritis, had little effect on concomitant prostatitis. There are no reports that such antibiotic therapy, when combined with regular prostatic massage, offers anything better. The fact that prostatitis, as defined, may be pre-existent and continue after the N.S.U. is cured, emphasizes the difficulty of placing the diagnosis on a scientific basis. The part played by such physiological phenomenon as the peri-prostatic blood congestion, which so commonly prompts early morning penile erection, in effecting passage of white cells into the prostatic secretions cannot be ignored. To pose the question, therefore, as to whether the presence of many white cells in prostatic secretion is physiological or pathological continues to be justifiable.

Treatment of N.S.U. is generally effective with one of the tetracycline group of antibiotics. Some physicians use streptomycin by injection, together with oral sulphonamides, as their first choice. Other antibiotics have also been used. In some men the condition proves difficult to control and the antibiotics may have to be employed on a trial-and-error basis. As in gonorrhoea, repeated follow-up examinations and tests are essential to full care and reassurance. It is customary to check prostatic secretion at three months from the presumed time of infection.

Relapse and recurrence occurs in at least 10 per cent of men within five years. The reasons are not always clear. Latent prostatitis is suspected in some. In others the 'virus' is thought to reassert itself after a period of latency in much the same way as the virus of 'cold sores' declare their presence from time to time.

D

Over and above the local complications, some 3 per cent of men with N.S.U. develop what is known as Reiter's syndrome or disease, so called after the name of its second discoverer. The syndrome, a combination of signs and symptoms, includes the urethritis, together with arthritis, usually of more than one joint, and inflammation of the eyes. Some men also develop skin and mouth lesions. The whole syndrome may be acute, subacute or chronic. It is frequently recurrent. The syndrome, based on a sexually transmitted N.S.U., is commonest in this country and the United States. In other parts of the world the syndrome, including the urethritis, may follow an attack of bacillary dysentery, a bowel infection.

Acute attacks of Reiter's syndrome or disease may be relatively mild but on occasion they resemble acute rheumatic fever. The subacute and chronic varieties with their tendency to flare up may resemble other forms of arthritis, such as spondylitis and rheumatoid arthritis. Loss of work for weeks or months is frequent in young men with the acute form. In the subacute and chronic cases recrudescences of the disease may lead to considerable degrees of crippling, particularly of the spine and feet. Impaired vision from recurrent inflammatory attacks in the eyes is also a threat. Blindness has been reported, as has involvement of the heart.

Many theories have been advanced to explain the cause of Reiter's arthritis and its associated phenomena. None, however, has stood up to critical examination. The one which forms the basis for rational treatment is that the condition is primarily an infectious urethritis to which some men, and occasionally women, react in an unusual way. There is some evidence that such people may be predisposed by heredity to this type of irregular reaction, as happens in other forms of 'rheumatism'. The classical parallel is the streptococcal throat infection, which is followed after an interval of two or three weeks by an attack of acute rheumatism, with high fever and joint pains and swelling. Treatment based on this theory therefore aims at clearing the urethritis, or 'trigger', as soon as possible, with antibiotics or sulphonamides or a combination of both. So far there is no indication that the non-specific urethritis of Reiter's syndrome is different from the more usual form of such cases. Concomitant and subsequent treatment of the arthritis and its accompaniments by appropriate measures, with rest and medication, will relieve pain, the most prominent element. Occasionally fever therapy, cortisone and/or splinting of affected joints is required.

In all cases of N.S.U. it has become customary to recommend examination and sometimes treatment of the affected man's wife or consort. The standard clinical and laboratory examinations and tests reveal a variety of conditions. In essence these findings are no different from those that are found in a comparable control group of women. Non-specific changes are common in the human cervix. Such a condition is generally called an 'erosion'. No distinctive evidence of a type associated solely with N.S.U. is generally accepted as a clinical entity. So far the same may be said about urethritis in women. The indication for any treatment is therefore almost exclusively epidemiologically based. The treatment advised is usually identical to that which has effected cure of the male's urethritis. The value of this empirical treatment, by way of preventing complications in the woman and any children she may subsequently bear, is unknown; nor is there any proof that it prevents recurrence of N.S.U. in the husband or regular sexual partner. Two small series of identical treatment of involved couples showed no difference in the subsequent history of the men when compared with controls.[92, 73] So far no contrary view has been expressed.

In summary then, N.S.U. is a great 'nuisance' disease, both at the epidemiological and individual level. Incomplete understanding of its basic cause breeds doubts and anxiety and bedevils treatment. It is a source therefore of much heartache and domestic misery. The complication of Reiter's arthritis with the eventual possibility of crippling is the greatest single hazard to which a promiscuous male exposes himself today.

*

Much more common than urethral discharge in men is pathological vaginal discharge in women. Commoner by far than all
the other varieties of such discharge is trichomonal vaginitis.
The cause of this condition is the trichomonas vaginalis, a
microscopically small one-celled animal, little bigger than a
white blood cell (see Figure 6). It is one of a family of flagellated
protozoa, the most notable members including one which is
part-cause of black-head disease in turkeys; and another, well-
known in animal husbandry to cause vaginitis in cattle. Many
cows in a herd were, in days gone by, infected by the local bull.
They frequently aborted and became sterile. To the expense of
treatment of his cows, the farmer had to add loss of calves. In
the absence of any satisfactory treatment for the bull, the
animal had to be destroyed. Slaughter and artificial insemina-
tion have almost completely eradicated the disease in cattle.
Similar measures have not been advocated for humans!

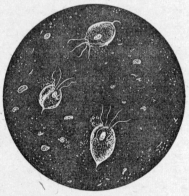

Figure 6. Specimen of vaginal discharge showing trichomonas vaginalis

The trichomonas with which we now concern ourselves is one
of five trichomonads capable of infesting man only. In the
human female its normal habitat is the vagina. More rarely it is
found in the urethra and neighbouring small glands. It does not
live in the rectum or the mouth. In men it may be found under

the foreskin, in the urethra and, on occasion, in secretion expressed from the prostate gland. Not unnaturally the parasite can sometimes be found in the urine.

Trichomonas vaginalis is most readily identified in wet specimens examined by the special dark-ground microscope technique. Recognition by staining methods is less satisfactory. The parasite can be cultivated in the laboratory without too much difficulty. It travels well and stays alive for two or three days in the same type of transport medium as that used for the organism of gonorrhoea.

The incidence of positive findings in women varies widely according to selection of groups for testing and the methods of diagnosis. Table 5 gives some idea of the variations. In an unselected group, if such a one exists, the figure would be about 20 per cent. Thus in England and Wales, we may conclude, over a million women, mostly in the sexually active age range, harbour the parasite. No age is immune, but it is unusual to find trichomonas vaginalis in those past the menopause and in those who have not yet reached puberty.

Trichomonas vaginalis is more commonly found in the pregnant than the non-pregnant and more often in coloured than in white women. It appears to be commoner in the lower socio-economic groupings and in the promiscuous. Some 50 per cent of women with gonorrhoea are found to suffer some degree of trichomonal vaginitis. Indeed, so often are the two conditions coexistent that many venereologists consider the presence of the trichomonas one of the medical indications for a search for gonococci.

Many women harbour the parasite with no complaint of symptoms, but trichomonas vaginalis is by far the commonest cause of pathological vaginal discharge. The condition, especially in younger women, may be acute and fulminating, with profuse and purulent vaginal discharge and irritation. Sanitary pads or tampons, used to stem the flood of discharge, are liable to become sodden and to add further irritation, discomfort and frank soreness. In other women, the complaint of vaginal discharge may be of some duration, often dating from a pregnancy,

Table 5 – Incidence of trichomonas vaginalis in various female groups

	T.V.+ percentage
Whittington (1951). Rural area.[112]	
562 Women attending a birth control clinic	5·3
507 Controls	3·4
55 Gynaecological patients	23·6
Whittington (1957). London Hospital[113]	
400 Gynaecological clinic patients	12·8
400 V.D. clinic patients	21·3
Feo (1956). America[28]	
301 Negro women attending medical clinic	12·3
439 White women attending medical clinic	2·9
74 Negro girls (10–19 years)	18·4
84 Negro girls (1–9 years)	3·6
Peter (1957)[85]	
1,300 Infants up to 1 year of age	1·0
Buxton et al. (1958)[12]	
465 married } insurance	6·3
single } clerks	1·4
575 Private gynaecological patients	6·9
715 Mental patients	15·0
221 Women prisoners	70·0
157 Undergraduates (20–22 years)	Nil
Burch et al. (1959). Washington D.C.[10]	
1,848 Health institute employees	17·7
Wang and Hsia (1958). China[108]	
1,460 Cotton millworkers	31·3
Verheye (1956). Congo[107]	
1,497 Presumably healthy women	27·0

months or years previously. The discharge in such cases is usually moderate in amount. It is sometimes malodorous. A slight degree of urethritis may accompany the vaginitis, and the parasite may linger in local glands. How often the parasite reaches the Fallopian tubes is not known. It has certainly been found there. Fortunately human trichomoniasis, as it is sometimes called, is not a recognized cause of abortion, miscarriage or sterility in women.

Cervical cytology, the method of examining specially stained scrapings of the cervix for cancer, is a common routine procedure whenever women are examined internally. Not infrequently the presence of trichomonas vaginalis is discovered by these tests. As a corollary, chronic trichomonal vaginitis causes changes in surface cells of the cervix, which may make the pathologist's task a difficult one. In such instances, as in any woman, the diagnosis of trichomonal infestation can easily be made by microscopic examination of a drop of the vaginal contents. Alternatively, and in addition, specimens may be prepared for culture tests.

Most men found to harbour the parasite in their genitourinary system have no symptoms. A few have urethritis. In a wide variety of studies using various diagnostic techniques, trichomonas vaginalis was found in 29–76 per cent, i.e. an average of half of the husbands or regular sex partners of women with the disease. Table 6 is reproduced from King's *Recent Advances in Venereology* and shows the findings from various parts of the world.[55]

Table 6 – *Trichomonas vaginalis in husbands or male consorts of women with trichomonal vaginitis*

		Cases		percentage T.V.+
Perl et al.	(1956)	48		58·0
Whittington	(1957)	24		33·3
Bedoya	(1957)	62		76·0
Dellapiane	(1957)	193		18·6
Keutel	(1959)	86		60·0
Burch et al.	(1959)	31		41·9
Block	(1959)	148	motile T. vaginalis	48·0
			non-motile T. vaginalis	13·5
Kostic	(1959)	364		39·0
Perju	(1959)	100		41·0
Rodin et al.	(1960)	38		29·0
Watt and Jennison	(1960)	30		60·0

The incidence in control series of men has varied from 0–8 per cent.

The other type of case is the man with non-gonococcal urethritis (N.G.U.) in whom trichomonas vaginalis is found. Estimates again vary in different series but the incidence is probably a little less than 5 per cent of all N.G.U. cases. In some, more especially those with an anatomical defect, whether congenital or acquired, the condition may be chronic and urethral discharge intermittent. The incubation period of trichomonal N.G.U. is probably between one and three weeks, and discharge is commonly accompanied by urethral irritation. Specimens for immediate microscopic and culture tests can be obtained from under the foreskin, from the urethra by gentle scraping with a fine wire loop, from the sediment of centrifuged urine and from prostatic secretion.

It will be noted that there is considerable disparity between the incidence figures of infestation in the sexes – around 20 per cent of women and probably less than 2 per cent of men. This difference does not seem to be accounted for solely by the problems of identifying the parasite in men, an admittedly difficult task. While the parasite may apparently inhabit the vagina for years without troublesome symptoms, similar chronicity in man is rarer; indeed, the natural course of events in the majority of infested men is for the parasite to disappear spontaneously after a few weeks. Experimental, clinical and laboratory evidence all support this view. Even crediting due allowance to these facts, some degree of unexplained disparity remains.

How the parasite is acquired is not always clear in the individual. Indirect methods of transmission such as transplantation of other human trichomonads, say from mouth or bowel to vagina, find no support in clinical or laboratory observations. Baths, bidets and swimming-pools are usually discounted since soap and chlorine are excellent trichomonacides. Further, the disease appears commonly in those less fastidious about personal hygiene, i.e., those who use such facilities less often. Towels have always seemed a possible source of infection but there is no information to support this view. The lavatory-seat theory is popular in some quarters. Whittington[113] arranged for thirty females known to be suffering from trichomonal vaginitis to use a W.C. Each patient found the lavatory seat in the 'up' position. When the seat was put 'down' a bell rang and informed Miss Whittington of the fact. The first observation to be made was that seventeen of the thirty patients were 'sitters' and thirteen 'non-sitters'. Of the first group, six left drops of discharge or urine on the front part of the seat. In three, T. vaginalis was found. Of the second group five left drops of discharge or urine and T. vaginalis was found in two. The parasite stays alive as long as the discharge is moist. Drying time not only depends on surrounding temperature but on the material of which the seat is constructed. Drying time may be as much as forty-five minutes. There is no doubt therefore that the parasite may find its way on to a lavatory seat and may live there for a time, but how does it find its way off, and can it accomplish this feat in the time available?

Another piece of research work recently reported concerns the possibility that T. vaginalis may be acquired from splashes arising when faeces is dropped into the contaminated water of a lavatory pan.[11] Through a hole in a piece of paper covering a lavatory seat, artificial faeces was dropped, and splashes on the underside of the paper counted. Distance from paper to water level was measured in a number of toilet arrangements and cistern-filling times noted. The relevance of these findings to the frequency of use of public conveniences was discussed. Women using such establishments are recommended by the researcher to flush the pan with the seat 'up' before use, as well as after. In this way contaminated splashes from the pan are minimized. Paper placed in the pan, after the first flushing, it is contended, would afford further immunity. Others recommended that all water closets for women should have seats with the front cut away.

Another source of indirect, and non-sexual, transmission appears to be the neo-natal period. This theory suggests that baby girls are infected by their mothers at birth and suffer a temporary vaginitis, the parasite then passing into a dormant phase, to reappear after puberty and give rise to symptoms. This theory has received scant attention in this country. Its basis lies in the fact that at birth, and for a few weeks thereafter, babies carry an accumulation of their mothers' sex hormones in the blood. These have the effect of making babies' breasts prominent. In baby girls the hormones also cause the vaginal lining and its secretions to be temporarily of the adult type – an ideal nidus for the support and reproduction processes of trichomonads. With the falling off of hormone levels within two or three weeks, it seems just possible that the parasite takes on a cystic or hibernating form and so exists till, at puberty, the girl, in providing her own sex hormones, recreates the ideal conditions.

That mothers can infect their baby daughters is not doubted by some researchers. Shaw,[97] for example, suggested this with his finding that thirty-six of forty-four virgin daughters of twenty-five mothers with trichomonal vaginitis harboured the parasite. More direct evidence comes from a Polish investigation[62] in which 2,006 girls aged from 0 to 17 years were examined for the presence of vaginal trichomonads. Of the girls aged 10–17 years, 10·4 per cent showed positive results ; 0·8 per cent of those aged 3 weeks to 10 years, and 17·2 per cent of 35 infants aged 0 to 3 weeks. This last group is admittedly small, but the findings are striking. They certainly indicate the need for a study with a family approach.

The fact and theory of neo-natal infection would help to explain the discrepancy in sexual distribution of the disease. It would also help to explain why trichomonal vaginitis is relatively common in young girls after what appears to be their first intercourse. The condition called 'honeymoon cystitis' is often an acute trichomonal vaginitis. It is suggested that local trauma, fluctuating hormone levels and psychic changes all contribute to a re-awakening of the parasite and the development of a pathological state.

While the possibility of indirect methods of transmission and precipitating factors can usefully explain a minority of cases, there is little doubt that the majority of women and probably all men infested with trichomonas vaginalis acquire the parasite during sexual intercourse. This was the general opinion of two major conferences on the subject – one at Rheims in 1957 and the other in Montreal in 1959. Since, however, the trichomonas may exist in women for years, the infecting intercourse, if there was one, may well be remote and forgotten when the diagnosis comes to be made. Many of the points already mentioned may be cited in support of sexual transmission. These, together with the fact that somewhere around half the husbands of infested women harbour the parasite and that, in the converse case, 100 per cent of wives or regular girl-friends of infested men are found with it,[17] places this view beyond reasonable doubt as operative in the majority of cases.

Modern treatment, with tablets by mouth, has revolutionized the outlook for sufferers from this common disease.[53] The new drug is called metronidazole. Cure is effected by a week's course of tablets in at least 80 per cent of the infested. Re-treatment effects cure in all. This applies to both sexes.

Some thought must be given to care of the asymptomatic husband of an infested woman. There would appear to be four possibilities. To do nothing about him precludes acceptance of the generally held view of sexual transmission. It invites recurrence of the vaginitis, although in practice this does not seem to happen very often. To treat the husband by proxy pays tacit allegiance to sex transmission but may well precipitate domestic discord, if in fact the wife interests the husband sufficiently to persuade him, in the absence of symptoms, to take his share of the tablets. A third method is to examine and treat all husbands irrespective of the findings. Each will require to be reassured regarding the absence of venereal disease. Husbands seem to accept the logic of investigation and epidemiological treatment. The fourth possibility is to investigate husbands and treat only those found to be infested. At the present there is no clear-cut evidence as to the best course to be followed. There would appear to be an obligation on those with the best facilities for diagnosis and full-scale laboratory follow-up to determine, by research, what is to be accepted as best for the patient.

As in other sexually transmitted diseases, follow-up examinations and tests are an integral part of the care of the couple.

Another common condition in women is moniliasis, or vaginal thrush. The fungus concerned in this condition is the same as that implicated in the oral thrush of babies, usually acquired by them from contaminated feeding bottles.

Fungus is a normal vaginal inhabitant of 20 per cent of women. Only in a small percentage, however, does it give rise to symptoms. The usual complaint is of vaginal discharge with irritation. Warmth aggravates the condition. Thus a woman begins to itch just when she is settling to sleep. In the worst instances, sleep may be seriously upset. A woman so pre-occupied night after night with scratching, soon suffers in appearance and temper. In pregnancy, when the condition is common, the white curd-like discharge may be widespread over the vaginal walls and the vulva. Fortunately symptoms arise in pregnancy much less often than might be expected. The presence of thrush in men, either as an affection under the foreskin, or as a form of urethritis, is rare.

A wide variety of fungicidal compounds is available either as paints or pessaries. The best of these are capable of controlling the condition in a few days.

Several skin conditions may affect the genitals. Not least amongst these is scabies, or 'the itch', caused by a tiny mite which burrows through the skin and which may be transferred from one person to another during sexual intercourse or where bed or blankets are shared. Similarly, crab lice may transfer themselves, to lay their eggs or nits, from the pubic hair – their natural habitat – of one person to that of another during coitus. Both of these skin conditions tend to show levels of incidence which parallel, at a low level, that of gonorrhoea.

Warts, viral in origin and thus infectious, tend to grow more readily and luxuriantly in warm and moist areas of the body. They may be found therefore under the foreskin in men and around the vaginal opening and the anus in women and more especially in those women with chronic vaginal discharge.

Cold sores or herpes, common around the mouth and nose, tend to appear where skin meets mucus membrane at the body's various orifices. The penis is a common site. Like cold sores elsewhere, the condition here is typified by recurrent attacks. It appears that the virus is acquired early in life and declares its presence from time to time for reasons that are not always clear. The condition can occur in women, around the vaginal opening, but is certainly rarer.

The term balanitis simply means inflammation under the foreskin. The common variety usually indicates lack of hygiene but may on occasion prophesy diabetes by some years.

Perfectly normal degrees of anxiety, amounting to no more than prudent caution, prompt many people to seek reassurance after casual sexual exposure.

Clinical examination and blood testing, repeatedly, if necessary, are generally sufficient for the doctor to give a confident word of reassurance to such people and for them to be satisfied.

There are, however, some in whom fears are more deeply rooted. They are people in whom the pressures of living become overwhelming and are transformed into symptoms. In the course of life they intermittently present the same symptoms or complain about a particular body system. The genito-urinary system bears its share. Thus, for example, many who learned bladder control but slowly, and who continued as bed-wetters into late childhood and even adolescence, form a recognizable group with somatic symptoms of a disturbed psyche. Symptoms, referrable to this and other systems of the body, frequently act as indicators and introductory gambits directing attention to real problems.

Anxiety to the point of panic, and sometimes mixed with remorse, dismay and shame, is not at all unusual in those who have exposed themselves to the possibility of infection. Fortunately, for the benefit of soul and psyche, confession and free discussion do good. Continued anxiety is more serious. It may be the earliest manifestation of serious depression and indicate the need for the expert assistance of a psychiatrist. For such sufferers the outlook today has never been better.

In some, guilt is the predominating manifestation of psychological disturbance. Like other symptoms, it may respond to one or several attendances for simple psychotherapy. Sometimes the degree of guilt is disproportionate to the act. It may be entirely ill-founded, and fear of infection may reach obsessional levels. Clearly such patients are in need of the most skilled and experienced psychiatric help.

In 1964 over 43,000 people attending special clinics in England and Wales were reported as 'not requiring treatment'. This is about 20 per cent of the total number of new patients. In this classification are many who required one or repeated consultations to secure complete reassurance or to re-establish their emotional equilibrium.

In this connexion, it is worth considering the role of information or propaganda about venereal and other sexually transmitted diseases. Kite and Grimble,[60] psychiatrist and venereologist respectively, caution against the fears that may be precipitated by disseminating such information. They call for all public discussion about venereal diseases to be sober, factual and free from moral overtones. With this few would disagree, but it does not provide a guarantee against mis-interpretation. Like children, the emotionally disturbed and readily unbalanced are liable to be highly selective in what they take from their reading, cinema-going or televiewing. That a few may be disturbed emotionally should be acceptable. Fear for the minority should not deny enlightenment to the many.

This chapter ends the descriptions of the diseases as they are seen and suffered in this country and throughout the world. I have had much in mind the young man who wrote to the *Guardian* in mid 1964, pointing out that nowhere could he find up-to-date information about these diseases in a lucid, lay form. The aim has been to match this challenge, without spreading alarm and despondency. At the risk of causing confusion, I have had to express inconclusive views, reflecting medical limitations. They give some hint of more serious problems in venereology both medical and social, and it is to these, as they present in a wide variety of ways, that we will now turn our attention.

7 Venereal Diseases as a Social Problem

Discussing this country's almost uninterrupted prosperity and peace during the century since Waterloo, Nicol,[80] writing under the heading 'Venereal Diseases – Moral Standards and Public Opinion', stated, 'But for the "have nots" of society, there was a darker picture of poverty, ignorance, disease and suffering, the price paid for the scientific advances of the industrial revolution.'

What price are we paying for today's prosperity, peace and technological revolution? Certainly not, in Britain at least, poverty and ignorance. On every hand affluence declares itself, particularly in clothing, feeding, travel and domestic and factory mechanization and automation. The 'have nots' are few. Education is free to all and compulsory up to 15 years of age. More and more children stay, voluntarily, longer and longer at an increasing array of schools, and our expanding university and technological institutions together with mass media have dispensed education, culture and facts with unprecedented lavishness. The price we pay today is therefore not poverty and ignorance. On both counts we could claim a credit balance. When we consider disease and suffering, however, all that can be claimed is a change of emphasis. The death-dealing fevers of infancy and childhood, and tuberculosis, that 'captain of the men of death', have been all but mastered. Other old menaces are being subjected to man's control. For example, the ravages of industrial diseases, malnutrition, the permanent asylum state of many mentally ill people, the blindness of the venereal diseases, the miseries of slum filth and smoke, overcrowding and child labour have gone or are going. In their place we have the deaths and deformities from an increasing number of road accidents; the epidemic of lung cancer; new levels of suicide and attempted suicide; excessively high rates of illegitimacy; vice, violence and delinquency in numbers hitherto unknown; increasing convictions for drunkenness; and child cruelty – together with uncontrolled levels of venereal disease. All these show something of the debit side of today's social balance sheet (see Table 7).

Table 7 – Incidence of some social phenomena in England and Wales

	1960	1961	1962	1963
All offences	1,035,212	1,152,397	1,266,596	1,319,147
Juveniles found guilty (a)	107,000	120,198	120,947	128,394
Wounding and assault	9,689	10,863	11,362	12,216
Cruelty to children	686	788	876	675
Breaking and entering	31,823	36,240	42,760	47,249
Brothel keeping	135	169	146	163
Prostitution offences	2,785	2,281	2,516	1,982
Charges for drunkenness	65,170	71,614	80,798	79,598
Suicides	5,113	5,200	5,588	5,715
Attempted suicides (b)	Estimated to be 6–8 times suicide rate			
Deaths from heart disease	142,258	146,007	150,611	154,815
Deaths from lung cancer	22,000	22,810	23,779	24,434
Legitimate births	742,000	746,445	767,354	795,000
Illegitimate births	43,000	48,000	55,000	59,000
Consumption of spirits (c)	15	16	16	17
Vehicles with current licence (thousands) (d)	9,384	9,907	10,505	11,384
Total casualties (d)	347,551	349,767	341,696	356,179
Deaths in road accidents (d)	6,970	6,908	6,709	6,912
Divorce – petitions filed	27,870	31,124	33,818	36,385
decrees absolute	23,369	24,936	28,376	31,405
Gonorrhoea	33,770	37,107	35,438	36,049

(a) Under 17 years. (b) See Stengel.[99] (c) Million Proof Gallons. (d) Great Britain.

Compiled mostly from the *Annual Abstract of Statistics* (1964), H.M.S.O., London.

From this jungle of sociological data let us turn to an examination of those factors inseparably associated with the venereal diseases. All types of people acquire infection but some of them can be seen to fall into recognizable groups. I propose to consider differing rates of infections in the sexes, the influence of age in infection, the problems of promiscuity and prostitution, and the part played by migrants and homosexuals. Not only will we try to see man in, as it were, social space, but we will try to define what can be recognized of his immediate social constellation at the time of infection. Thus we shall concern ourselves not only with the background to infection but with its social significance and effects.

No rank, social class, or profession provides immunity from venereal disease. Statistical data on the subject are of little value because at present they concern themselves with very local series of patients. I have already said that the number of infected men generally exceeds that of women. In the case of gonorrhoea, ratios vary from 2:1 to 6:1, but are usually 3–4:1. The ratio for syphilis is much nearer 2:1, since syphilis is more generally acquired from a regular contact and contacts can be more readily traced.

In recent years, with rising rates of infection, ratios have widened. A W.H.O. report on the position in England, Wales and Scotland[120] shows that racial factors may play some part. In the case of U.K.-born patients with gonorrhoea the ratio was 2·1:1, and for syphilis (under 1 year's duration) 4·2:1. For West Indian patients during the same period the ratios were gonorrhoea 8·4:1; syphilis 0·9:1; and for other immigrants 8·9:1 and 10·7:1. These striking racial differences may be accounted for by such associated factors as varying degrees of promiscuity, help given with the tracing of contacts, homosexuality, and possibly immunity from syphilis conferred on immigrants from yaws areas of the world.

Special attention has lately been paid to the age of those infected. Not unnaturally all are in the sexually active years. Girls mature, physically, earlier than boys and earlier than in less prosperous days. This, and the freedom which they enjoy equally with boys nowadays, is reflected in the incidence of disease. This is most readily noticeable in the most sensitive indicator of infection – gonorrhoea. Leslie Watt,[110] working in Manchester, reviewed the trends between 1938 and 1960. He noted the increase in adolescent venereal disease to be five times greater in U.K.-born girls than in U.K.-born boys. His figures were 25 per cent and 4·9 per cent respectively. Due allowance was made for the total numbers 'at risk', and repeat infections were excluded. The emphasis on youthful infections has been greatest in recent years. The British Co-operative Clinical Research Group,[7] reporting in 1960, found a 13·8 per cent increase in gonorrhoea in England and Wales between 1957 and 1958. The increase was most marked in the age group 15–19 years with the female contribution in that range increased by no less than 27·9 per cent. The Group looked at the question of differential increases more closely in their 1962 report.[8] For the years 1957–60, the distribution of further increases of gonorrhoea was as follows:

Males	15–19 years	–	67·3 per cent
	20–24 years	–	65·2 per cent
	Others	–	33·5 per cent
Females	15–19 years	–	65·4 per cent
	20–24 years	–	60·9 per cent
	Others	–	18·0 per cent

The trend continued through 1961 and 1962 and may be expressed in another way:

In 1961	Males	15–19 years formed	6·3 per cent of total
In 1962	Males	15–19 years formed	7·0 per cent of total
In 1961	Males	20–24 years formed	27·1 per cent of total
In 1962	Males	20–24 years formed	30·2 per cent of total
In 1961	Females	15–19 years formed	25·8 per cent of total
In 1962	Females	15–19 years formed	24·5 per cent of total
In 1961	Females	20–24 years formed	37·6 per cent of total
In 1962	Females	20–24 years formed	38·6 per cent of total

It will be remembered that the incidence of gonorrhoea fell slightly in 1962 and this was reflected in the figures for younger girls. Nevertheless girls aged 15–19, who form only 6·4 per cent of the female population, contributed 39·2 per cent of the female gonorrhoea in the years 1958–61. This is five times the increase in males of corresponding age.[8] According to Michael Scofield,[95] by the age of 18 twice as many boys as girls have had intercourse. His findings were 34 per cent and 17 per cent respectively. In general boys have a greater number of consorts. Nevertheless the chances of a girl becoming infected are about 1 in 1,000 and of a boy 1 in 1,600. He gave as the reason for this apparent discrepancy the finding that there is a restricted number of girls who are highly promiscuous.

As from the year 1963 the Ministry of Health has sought information from clinics in England and Wales regarding the ages of patients. For 1963[89] the figures show that of 7,446 women and girls with gonorrhoea, 2,060 (27·6 per cent) were aged 19 years and under. The trend therefore continues and must be considered grave.

The last word on this topic should go to Lord Stoneham, Joint Parliamentary Under Secretary of State to the Home Office, who, pointing out in 1964 that the matter was of considerable concern, stated that in the preceding six years cases of gonorrhoea in the 15–24 age group had increased by more than 60 per cent in boys and nearly 80 per cent among girls.[91]

Similar trends are reported from the U.S.A., Sweden and Finland. In Denmark[78] the increase in gonorrhoea has been extensively analysed in girls under 25. The increase is both absolute and relative. Those in the age range 15–19 constituted 19·5 per cent of all infected women in 1944. In 1961 they comprised 43 per cent; that is to say, about 1 in 100 of all Danish girls in this age range was infected during one calendar year.

Much that is yet ill-understood lies behind the type of teenage female behaviour which brings about a substantial proportion of these figures in this country and elsewhere. The starting-point is often teenage revolt, which takes the form of staying out later and later, against orders sometimes. Eventually the girl stays out all night and, without warning, goes missing. She becomes a roamer. This is predominantly a female activity, as pointed out in Mary Ellison's book *Missing from Home*.[26] For many girls running away from home is the final step in revolt and the first in social decline. Many become promiscuous. Some of the men concerned are charged with having unlawful intercourse because the girls are, in fact, below 16 years of age. Many of the girls become diseased, and help to form the female reservoir of infection.

What sort of girl breaks down socially in this way and why? Writing under the heading of 'The Road to Promiscuity', J. O'Hare,[83] a woman medico-social worker at the Department of Venereology in St Mary's Hospital, London, stated that 86 out of 100 promiscuous* girls under 20 came from financially secure homes where the family provided all material comforts and needs. What the girls did lack in the home or from the local boys was their own idea of interest and affection. They grew impatient of restraint, discipline and boredom. They craved independence and freedom and instant satisfaction of every whim. They began to live only for the moment.

With many of the girls it was difficult to decide whether or not they were prostitutes. They were all clear in their own minds that they were not. About 50 per cent of them associated with itinerant males, who constitute an attractive target for the dissatisfied girl seeking demonstrative affection. Men of a different nationality offered special glamour. The writer concludes from her study:

The promiscuous spring from every class of society and every type of home. Lack of an intelligent and affectionate approach by the parents is a pre-disposing factor. Society in general, by refraining from moral sanctions, has smoothed the path which is made more attractive and brought forcibly and persistently to notice, by business interests. Films, the Press, dress and cosmetic firms all concentrate on the importance of sexual attraction. But for every girl impelled to

* Promiscuity is defined in the *Oxford English Dictionary* as 'indiscriminate mixing'. How many sex contacts – and in what space of time – a person must have to be labelled 'promiscuous' has never been defined.

promiscuity by these external factors a girl can be found in precisely similar circumstances who has resisted them, the individual character and psychological make-up being the final determining factor.

This last point was taken up by others. Ponting reported on 200 girls aged 13–20 from Leeds and London.[86] She saw the high incidence of V.D. in them as but one symptom of the altered manners of young people. Although 25 per cent had a grammar-school place, they, like their less gifted sisters, rarely made full use of their educational opportunities. Their job records showed a tendency to drift and few had any training. Many came from 'good homes' in which, however, individual family members tended to go their separate ways. The family as a unit shared very few outings and activities. In all but nine, father appears as a nonentity.

Elizabeth Keighley[54] believed from her studies of 107 girls aged 16–19, almost all of them on remand, that immaturity was common amongst them. She used as her criteria of maturity in a girl the ability to fulfil at least three of the following requirements:

1. Good work record.
2. Fondness of home activities and/or some constructive spare-time interest.
3. A steady male relationship without promiscuity.
4. Some realization of future actions and where these should lead.
5. An ability to see present circumstances and background with some detachment and/or (where there has been a family background) in some sense of responsibility to the family.

By these criteria 96 girls were judged immature. Regression to childlike behaviour is of course common in both physical and emotional illness. To find it in those who have broken down socially is perhaps not surprising. How much, in these cases, preceded, and how much followed break-down is not determined. What does seem definite and alarming is the form of expression taken by the immaturity. I should make clear at this point that in the opinion of myself and others these girls' indulgence in sexual activity is rarely motivated by any biological urge for orgasm. Sexual activity culminating in orgasm is nearly unknown among them. Their need for a man is social rather than sexual. Each girl has a need to show both herself and her peers that she can command what a grown woman commands. To prove herself a woman she may find it necessary to become pregnant. To say that such girls have unwanted pregnancies is, if we confine ourselves to the girls' mental state before conception, to misjudge their needs. In other words, the pregnancies are wanted.

How far along the road to promiscuity is the turning marked 'Prostitution'? The answer is not always clear. Indeed it is often a matter of definition. A prostitute, or as she may prefer to be called, 'a business girl', is certainly one who takes money, but what of the girl who for kind rather than cash has intercourse with a variety of men? Many of these girls would not consider themselves prostitutes and many self-regarding prostitutes call them 'tarts' or 'whores', terms loaded with invective and used with the same vehemence as the militant trade unionist uses 'blackleg'. Most reports from abroad consider only financial involvement in their definition, but in this country both those who take money and those who practise sex promiscuously, in exchange for beer, food, clothing or a roof for the night, are frequently included. With this precautionary note in mind, we can say that the incidence of prostitution and the contribution it makes towards the incidence and spread of venereal disease varies with both time and place. In Africa and Asia and parts of South America, the prostitute has been, and continues to be, the source of at least 80 per cent of infection. In Asia especially the prostitute is tolerated and to some extent highly organized. In spite of this, or because of it, she is often infectious. In Europe, and especially in France, Italy and Spain, there has tended to be a two-standard arrangement, that is, organized prostitution side by side with the chaperonage system. This has in the past certainly provoked a dual morality – on the one hand that brothels are a necessity and on the other that some women are too good for sex. Between these extremes a wide spectrum of views existed. These have tended to prevail. The organized brothel with its police registration of prostitutes and regular medical inspections (often never adequate, and frequently perfunctory) has given way to clandestine prostitution as exemplified by the street-walker. In the continental countries mentioned, and elsewhere, chaperonage is now rarer and the regular girl-friend with pre-marital sex experience is common.

Something of these changing European views and practices can be seen from enactments in France. Registered prostitution was long recognized in that country. In 1940 all prostitutes were forced to have regular medical examinations and, if necessary, treatment. Compulsory notification of infection was introduced in 1942. In 1946 the emphasis was on the diseased prostitute as the source of much, if not most, of the post-war peak rates of infection. The licensed brothels were closed and licensed street-walking was abolished. Public reaction was, in general, fierce. Severe penalties were imposed, for example, in cases of procurement. All this led to a great increase in clandestine and part-time prostitution.[109]

The Merlin law of February 1958 closed the houses of prostitution in Italy. The first report of the working of the law appeared in 1960. Among a long list of its medical and social 'failures' was noted an increase in uncontrolled provincial prostitution and venereal disease.[33] Another pointer to the dangers of uncontrolled prostitution comes from Japan,[114] in an article dated 1962. When 1,970 prostitutes were examined 10·7 per cent of those from controlled houses were found to have gonorrhoea, as against 42·2 per cent among uncontrolled street-walkers.

In this country street-walking prostitutes have long prevailed, and have presented problems. In the late 1950s the so-called clandestine nature of their professional activities all but ceased. Many of our large city centres became parade grounds for the most blatant plying of trade. Dr Elizabeth Keighley[52] examined 387 prostitutes in Holloway gaol, London, during 1958. No less than 145 (37 per cent) were aged 15–20. Seventy-one (48·9 per cent) of these girls had gonorrhoea. They accounted for more than half the total number of cases found. The law of the time demanded evidence of annoyance of passers-by before an arrest could be made. 'Fines only' was the order of the day, with maximum of forty shillings for the first and all subsequent offences. This was a trivial amount to the average street-walker or her ponce. Clearly, the law was not only an ass but manifestly appeared to be so. Following the *Report of the Committee on Homosexual Offences and Prostitution* (the Wolfenden Report), the Street Offences Act of 1959 became law. For the convicted prostitute, scaled fines, up to £25, can now be ordered, with or without periods of imprisonment. Long terms of imprisonment fall on those found guilty of living on immoral earnings.

These repressive measures have been effective in clearing the streets of our big cities. The social stigma of parading prostitutes both by day and night has been removed. Not so prostitution. The effects of the Act on the incidence of gonorrhoea was only locally and temporarily beneficial. Prostitutes largely re-organized their activities to make their pick-ups in pubs, cafés and clubs, and perhaps with more discretion in the streets. In 1963 at Holloway gaol, when, for the first time in several years, there was a fall in the number of prostitutes, 415 were seen. Of these, 85 (20 per cent) were aged 15–20. Of all the girls examined, 20 per cent had gonorrhoea and 1·9 per cent had syphilis; 39 were pregnant.[89]

As prosperity sweeps the Western world there is of course less economic pressure or necessity for women and girls to become prostitutes. The basic necessities are available to all who care to work, and work is plentiful. What is 'necessary' is, however, relative to us all and perhaps more so to many young and often immature and very impressionable females. Especially is this so in those apparently allergic to parental restraint and highly susceptible to advertising. Ready conformity to influence from their peers is another common feature of the behaviour that leads through promiscuity to overt prostitution. The 'oldest profession' therefore continues. As a prime cause of venereal disease it is, however, outstripped in this and other socially advanced and prosperous countries by the advent of the pro-miscuous or 'good-time' girl.

While admitting the limitations of definitions and the absence of controls it can be agreed, says Willcox,[114] that in France in recent years the prostitute has provided 25–34 per cent of the infections, while in the U.S.A. her contribution lies between 5–13 per cent. For this country the current figure is around 15–19 per cent which compares with the 35·7 per cent reported in our big cities for 1954[6] and Laird's[66] 34 per cent as taking cash, and 22 per cent as taking kind, in Manchester in 1958.

There have been few medico-social studies of prostitutes in this country. In 1955 Eleanor French[31] drew a picture of them from a close study of 150. She was at pains to point out that since all had landed in trouble, her study was therefore confined to 'failures'. She found most of the girls and women to be from poor social backgrounds and of average intelligence or less. They showed such minority group traits as lack of responsibility; a sense of being at war with the world; a propensity to lying, easily and pleasantly; being emotionally facile, even in their group loyalties, and sometimes proud of their frigidity. In some measure the prostitute was the female image of the male criminal. Of the 150 concerned, 64 were known to have associated with criminals. The writer went further:

> Not only is the link with crime a real one but there is an even darker side to the picture, for where prostitution exists among the wealthier sections of a community, it is inevitably tied up with vice and perversion and this must not be forgotten if we are to form a true picture of what prostitution involves. Prostitution is not legally a crime, any more than adultery or fornication, but it acts as a kind of magnet that attracts to itself the worst elements of society, the third party exploiter and the criminal. For this reason alone we cannot be indifferent to the problem it presents.

This was written in 1955 when the case of Stephen Ward was more than half a decade away.

In this context it is worth recollecting that it took international bodies from 1904 till 1949 to suppress finally what was colourfully called 'the white slave traffic' in girls. One body after another found that the greatest incentive to the trade was the organized brothel system. Glib-tongued men dangling the carrots of idle ease and glamour seem to have had little difficulty finding girls and women. How happily, or otherwise, and even how successfully, these women operated as prostitutes on behalf of their ponces is unknown.

By way of transition to a more detailed study of the male side of the social background of venereal diseases we might consider the type of men who form the prostitutes' clientèle. Little research has been done anywhere in this field. According to Kinsey[59] 34 per cent of single American men had had intercourse with a prostitute before the age of 25. How far this finding is applicable to men in this country at the present time is not known. Most observers would agree that it is near the truth for the generation who spent four to six years of their early manhood in the services during the last war.

Gibbens and Sibermann, a psychiatrist and a psychiatric social worker, interviewed 230 clients of prostitutes.[34] The great majority were between 20 and 40 years of age. By their bewildering variety of histories and personalities they seemed very near a representative cross-section of males of their age. If they had any group characteristics at all, these were that they tended to be passive men and were often of good general character. They tended to live at home with a dominant mother. Frequently father was dead or of equally little account. Only 15 per cent admitted intercourse with the same prostitute on more than one occasion. In only 15 per cent was a friendly relationship with the girl claimed.

More studies regarding male V.D. patients in general have been undertaken. Of particular interest are war-time studies in the American and Canadian armies. The American study suggests that promiscuity is related to an incapacity to form a deep attachment with one woman and has its origin in poor emotional adjustment. Like other phenomena of social significance it is common when morale is poor. No evidence of glandular defects which might increase sexual needs to unusual degrees was found. The Canadian army study of men infected with venereal disease classified them as the unstable, the heavy drinker, the immature and the dull. It was added that infection does not alter their habits. In this country Dalzell-Ward, Nicol and Haworth[22] conducted group discussions with male V.D. patients. Two points came out clearly: most men in the groups cherished the belief that there are two types of women, good and bad. Secondly, they believed that sexual intercourse is necessary for health.

Migration appears to be high on the list of causes of a rising V.D. rate. This is especially so in recent years in the Western world. The immigrant population of continental Europe alone is now estimated at 3·5 millions. Multiracialism is rapidly becoming an established fact. Nearly one in four West Germans has come from the Eastern sector. The French population has been swelled by nearly a million from North Africa. Planned immigration of Indonesians into Holland is under way. In Switzerland one in six is an immigrant, many from Turkey and North Africa. The Swiss Government's decision to establish in the heart of Europe a hospital for tropical diseases leaves one in no doubt that the trend is expected to continue.

The increase in the problem of immigrants in this country has mainly concerned peoples from the Commonwealth, many of them from the West Indies. The 1961 census for England and Wales[18] places numbers at 686,422 and 171,796 respectively. This last figure compares with the 15,301 of 1951. The tenfold increase far outruns the 37 per cent increase of those from the Irish Republic (Eire) and the 39 per cent increase of those from Northern Ireland. The total increase in immigrants over the ten years was from 491,620 to just over 1·5 millions. This figure is of course a balance (as at April 1961) of all those who had come here and all those who had gone home again.

As in other countries, immigrants tend to concentrate in large cities where there are opportunities for living and mixing with their own people and where the chances of finding work and education are more plentiful. In this country, perhaps more so than elsewhere, the tendency has been to accept large numbers of unattached males, rather than to encourage families. Some, like the West Indians and the Irish, marry late or not at all. The

West Indians come from areas of the world with high promiscuity rates, judged by levels of illegitimacy and venereal disease. However, all are agreed that they do not as a rule arrive in this country in an infected state. (My own experience is that much more infection is imported by U.K.-born tourists returning from the continent.) For this reason, as well as others, proposals to examine immigrants for venereal infection as a routine at ports of entry is likely to be unhelpful in controlling or curbing rising syphilis and gonorrhoea rates.

All immigrants on arrival here are subject to the stresses and strains of homesickness and the problems of settling in a new land. They come from a wide variety of backgrounds. Their education and religion represent all levels and creeds. With the exception of the Irish and the West Indians, there are language difficulties. Colour may restrict full social acceptance. Like first-generation immigrants anywhere in the world, they tend to form a society within a society. The West Indian with his merry and adventurous spirit, generosity and command of English has many advantages over his brothers from elsewhere in the Commonwealth.[3] This has been delineated by Hall,[43] who emphasizes the restrictions here, regarding housing and recreational facilities. Others, in reviewing the social and sex habits of immigrants generally, have pointed out that a disproportionately small number of females and families have accompanied men from all parts of the Commonwealth. The lesson of history is that this is the very worst type of immigration, and calculated to end with trouble.

In spite of all their handicaps, however, our immigrants are well behaved if one compares them with soldiers of any nation stationed abroad. Immigrants seek the companionship of native-born women and tend to find them in pubs, clubs and cafés. Many of the girls are promiscuous and some are runaways, roamers or, as some call them, 'mysteries'. Not surprisingly, they are frequently infected. M. Mary Beveridge[3] has shown the pattern prevailing with the West Indian, who prefers to take his pick-up home to his flat. The Pakistani and Adenese, because of religious teaching, usually avoid pubs and alcohol and are often served by 'itinerant tarts' who call at their houses. These 'call girls' recognize that the religious scruples about alcohol and the language difficulties of many Moslem men severely curtail their social activities. These observations were made in Sheffield, but since then similar conditions have been reported from Bradford.

Some idea of the degrees of promiscuity prompted by these circumstances may be obtained when incidence figures are based ethnically. From the East End of London, King reported in 1958[56] the findings of the period November 1955–November 1956. Of 925 men seen with gonorrhoea, 219 (23·7 per cent) were West Indian and 304 (32·8 per cent) from other parts of the Commonwealth. From Manchester for the years 1956–7 Laird reported[66] that only 47 per cent of males with gonorrhoea were native-born. The others were divided as follows: West Indians 21 per cent; West Africans 12 per cent; men from the Irish Republic 13 per cent; other Europeans and Asians 7 per cent. Knight[61] reported from Birmingham for 1957. His gonorrhoea cases can be divided ethnically into: 'Whites' 40 per cent; West Indians 49 per cent; Indians and Pakistanis 10 per cent.

Figures are available at national level. By 1960, of 21,663 males with gonorrhoea (about 90 per cent of the reported total for England and Wales) only 49·5 per cent were born in the United Kingdom; 25·5 per cent in the West Indies and 25 per cent in other parts of the Commonwealth or elsewhere. The corresponding figures for 5,912 females were: 83 per cent U.K.-born; 7·9 per cent West Indian and 9·1 per cent others. By 1962 the trend was in the same direction with only 44 per cent of males with gonorrhoea native-born. Both the male and female West Indian contribution rose.[115] In the same report Willcox makes an analysis of the morbidity rates of the different ethnic groups. Using a Home Office estimate – no immigration figures are kept – of 250,000 West Indians (200,000 males and 50,000 females) he calculated their morbidity rate for 1961 at 4,029·5 infections per 100,000 per annum for males and 148·8 for females. (The 1961 census figure for West Indians was 171,786.) This is to be compared with the overall morbidity figure of

202·4 male infections and 75·5 female infections per 100,000 for the rest of the population. In a decade male immigrants were responsible for 54·2 per cent of the increase in male gonorrhoea, while U.K.-born females were responsible for 70·7 per cent of the total female increase. These two major elements, immigrants and U.K.-born females, although clearly connected, have some basic distinctions and divergencies of rates and trends which are not yet fully explained.

The Commonwealth Immigrants Act was introduced in the middle of 1962. It came at a time when rising, if patchy, unemployment was particularly affecting recently arrived immigrants. The general fall or levelling off of spending power was paralleled by a levelling off in the rising gonorrhoea rate during the second half of 1961 which continued into 1962. In this year the rate fell by 4·5 per cent and the group totals most affected were U.K.-born males, teenage females and West Indian males, in that order. The contribution made by the Commonwealth Immigrants Act to this reversal has been temporary. The 1963 figures[9] show a rise again, although at 1·6 per cent the curve of increase is flatter. The Act has reduced the number of immigrants entering the U.K. from around 100,000 per annum at the peak, to some 50,000 per annum since. Many have the impression that wives and families form a larger proportion than formerly. No figures are available of the number currently returning home. Of all the factors operating against control of gonorrhoea in this country, the promiscuity of immigrants is the most potent. Whether or not this will continue to play the leading role depends on the number of unattached males entering the United Kingdom. The waiting list of those seeking entry to the U.K. must at present be somewhere in the region of 300,000.

The increase in infections among U.K.-born males is not great. It does, however, underline that without immigration, the venereal infection rate would probably still have risen. In Scandinavian countries large-scale immigration is unknown, yet the rise there in the incidence of gonorrhoea has been amongst the most spectacular.

The immigrant is of course only one form of itinerant. Long

before the present problem of immigrants loomed so large on the social scene, itinerants generally were recognized as potential sufferers from infection. A report in 1956[6] showed that 40 per cent of all infected men acquired their disease with a casual contact, while away from home. Some have gone so far as to suggest that venereal infection is an occupational hazard of seamen of all nationalities, travellers and tourists generally, and long-distance lorry drivers in particular. Immigrants, with no home ties, are frequently itinerant within the land of their adoption, spending holidays or week-ends with friends or relatives in other cities. They show the same readiness to move when waves of unemployment strike. In all these instances the familiar figures of the V.D. scene are the mobile male and the static female. In recent years, both parties are frequently on the move and so 'at risk'. In the 'call girl' system already mentioned the usual picture is reversed.

Another minority group prone to social isolation and seeking integration has been more clearly delineated in recent years. Few developments in the epidemiological field of venereal disease have been more striking than the growth (both apparent and real in the opinion of many,) of male homosexuality. The growth of this phenomenon has been a feature of the literature of the last decade in several countries, including Denmark, France and the United States. Gonorrhoea and syphilis, and occasionally non-specific urethritis, are more commonly acquired in homosexual activity than ever before. It has been a matter of concern to venereologists that young homosexuals, especially, should be found ignorant of this fact.

The current situation in this country is well documented. At St Mary's Hospital, London, in the years 1954–56, only 12 per cent of early male syphilis cases occurred in homosexuals. In the years 1960–62 the figure was 65 per cent.[48] At St Thomas's Hospital, London, at the end of the last decade, some 13 per cent of men with gonorrhoea had acquired their disease homosexually. London is something of a magnet for homosexuals and those who attend provincial V.D. clinics have frequently spent

part of their working life in the Metropolis. In the provinces
only about 30 per cent of early male syphilis and 3 or 4 per cent
of male gonorrhoea is currently acquired homosexually. This is
higher than previously recognized. Confirmation of this trend is
reflected in the national ratio of male to female cases of syphilis.
The usual ratio over many years has been between 2:1 and 3:1.
In 1957, for instance, it was still 2·9:1. By 1961 it was 4·2:1.
Similar changes have been noted in the Rudolph Berg Hospital,
Copenhagen.[94] In 1961 some 25 per cent of fifty-two men with
early syphilis were homosexual. It was noted that the male to
female ratio of cases had changed from 1·1:1 in 1957 to 4·6:1 in
1961. This report also revealed that half of the homosexually
infected men did not seek advice, as the primary sore was elsewhere than on the genitals and its true nature not appreciated.

Kinsey[59] in his *Sexual Behaviour in the Human Male* (1948)
stated that 37 per cent of all American men had some overt
homosexual experience between adolescence and old age. Of the
white males in his series, 4 per cent were exclusively homosexual
throughout their lives. There was a general feeling in this
country at the time of publication of these figures that at least
the first was too high for application to men in the United
Kingdom. There is mounting evidence that both percentages
may be acceptable today. The whole subject of homosexuality
has been adequately, soberly and factually explored by West.[111]

For a view of the homosexual as seen in the venereal disease
clinic, Jefferiss' paper[48] will serve us well. He found, working in
London, that the overall incidence in his department was 8·4
per cent of all his male patients. Of 224 consecutive homosexuals, 164 had gonorrhoea; 10 syphilis; 16 non-specific
urethritis; and the others (15 per cent) had no apparent disease.
Their age range ran with that of his heterosexual patients. Clerical
and artistic trades and professions were prominent but all
classes were represented. Ninety-seven considered themselves
'passive', that is, they adopted the female role, while 127 were
'active'. Twenty-four styled themselves as 'versatile'. As might
be expected from this classification, ano-rectal and penile
disease was more or less equally distributed. The group's past

E

history of 15 per cent with previous venereal infection supports the general impression that many homosexuals are promiscuous. Of 54 men questioned at length, 40 (70 per cent) came from broken homes; 23 (42 per cent) had been brought up by mother only and 10 had never known either parent.

The discussion as to the parts played by genetic and environmental factors in determining male homosexuality has gone on for many years and it continues. In his conclusions, Jefferiss judged that of his 54 closely studied men, 51 were 'congenital' homosexuals, while 3 had 'acquired' this form of sexual expression. This conclusion is of interest in view of Kallman's recent work in America.[50, 51] Surmounting great difficulties he found 85 homosexually inclined twin men. Most of them were more or less entirely homosexual. Of the 85, forty were identical twins, i.e. from the same ovum as their brother and so not only identical in appearance but in all such respects as blood group, finger-prints, etc. Twins of 37 of these 40 men were traced by Kallman. He found that all of them could be rated homosexual, 28 of them exclusively so. These findings were in striking contrast to those in the non-identical twin group. Of 45 originals, 26 twin brothers were traced. Of these only 3 were homosexuals.

The Misses Green and Moore, who studied 33 male homosexuals[37] and reported eight years later than Jefferiss, had little new to add. They underlined the observation that homosexuality as seen in this country is almost exclusively confined to European stock. Others have made observations on the social aspects of the problem. Michael Schofield, research director of the Central Council for Health Education, believes that with no treatment available that is accepted as generally beneficial it may be forecast that present levels of homosexuality can be expected to persist. He sees no hope of a decrease. He believes that part of the problem, at present, is that men are more likely to admit their homosexuality and to practise it more freely since the Wolfenden Report brought a better informed and more sympathetic public view. Practising homosexuals, Schofield reminds us, are law-breakers, and it may be the inherent fear of authority which makes them relatively poor sources of sex contact information. The ratios of male to female cases of early syphilis already quoted do not seem to bear this out, and many venereologists would find the suggestion unacceptable.

Of all the definable factors involved in the spread of venereal disease, only one other has proved worthy of study. This is the role of alcohol. Even modest amounts are liable to impair a man's critical faculties, and such a state, in the presence of a prostitute or a practised promiscuous pick-up, all too frequently leads to unpremeditated exposure, with subsequent infection. About 30 per cent of infected men appear to meet their source of disease in a public-house. Although the total number of convictions for drunkenness has steadily increased in recent years (see Table 7) associated outright drunkenness is a less usual story with the venereally infected than ten or fifteen years ago. The tendency for the role of excess alcohol to decline as an adjuvant to infection has been pointed out by Beveridge.[3] She has shown that this is related to the increased proportion of immigrant patients. For linguistic and religious reasons the Pakistani and the Adenese usually eschew the public-house. The West Indian uses the pub more as a rendezvous or contact point and usually avoids an excess of alcohol. The present-day U.K.-born man, however, mixes his 'pleasures' and frequently suffers from both. The ancient ritual of 'taking a woman in his cups' persists apparently from the Saxon Ealuscerwen or ale terror. Those who would care to see how much better a husband than lover the Englishman makes, would do well to consult Nina Epton's *Love and the English*.[27]

The role of general socio-economic factors in the epidemiology of the venereal diseases is complex, and most authorities have shown caution in estimating their influence. The steady decline in syphilis since the middle of last century, although now being interrupted by another rise, has been attributed to the general spread of economic progress with better average living-standards. Some may question whether this explains the decline in syphilis behind the Iron Curtain. In the late 1950s we had the phenomenon in this and other thriving countries of declining syphilis rates alongside rising gonorrhoea rates. Now, while admitting a decline in syphilis with the economic depression of 1929–31, we find it again on the rise here and in other countries in spite of unprecedented levels of general prosperity. Gonorrhoea too, only recently classed by some as a 'dying disease', is as common as ever. All this applies particularly to countries showing unusually rapid economic progress, whether migration takes place to them or not. Migration for some countries is in fact a symptom of economic progress. As the children of Israel made for the 'promised land', so these of the underdeveloped countries make for lands of promise.

The contrast between the conditions in the countries of the Western world and those behind the Iron Curtain is striking. The state of affairs in Russia, for example, was studied by a W.H.O. team of twenty-two physicians from nineteen countries over a period of six weeks in 1961. They found that the general and world-wide decline in infectious syphilis had continued there uninterrupted. The official morbidity figures were given as 24·6 per 100,000 of the population in 1950 and 1·4 per 100,000 in 1960, when the level in England and Wales was 2·1 per 100,000 and rising. The success rate in the control of gonorrhoea was less spectacular: 81·36 per 100,000 in 1950 and a steady fall to 57·2 per 100,000 in 1960, when the rate in England and Wales was about 75 per 100,000 and rising. Routine tests for gonorrhoea are quite usual in many parts of Russia. How far these figures, and more especially their continuing decline, are due to routine measures in a widely spread network of 6,000 clinics; confidential but compulsory notification, as undertaken by 'patronage' nurses; and heavy penalties, for example, for homosexual offences, is a matter of speculation. While the Russian degree of economic development, at least at the personal level, has not matched that of many Western countries, the U.S.S.R. might well claim that steady socio-economic improvement, an efficient venereal disease service and widespread and continuous efforts in the educational field had all paid, and continued to pay, handsome dividends. How far and how thoroughly these facilities and measures would cope with Western-type prosperity and all that means in itinerancy, immigration, greater individual spending power, the advertising of the wares of free enterprise and the liberalism of teenage freedom, prostitution and homosexuality, will perhaps be revealed to the next or next but one generation.

It is not possible to leave the question of socio-economics and venereal diseases without making clear that wars, with their disruption of family and economic stability, have been the most potent encouragers of venereal diseases. They offer the 'doom' philosophy, like prosperity's 'boom' philosophy of eat, drink and be merry.

Peace, probably more often than war, offers unrivalled opportunities to study man in his changing environment. Something of such studies has been presented in this chapter, and it must now be apparent that the circumstances in which people are born, nurtured, mature and live will to some extent colour their conduct. For most, upbringing is a matter of acceptance or resignation. Some appear to live above their environment, while others are its victims. Clearly, then, from this and previous chapters, the problem of venereal disease, and to some extent other sexually transmitted diseases, emerges as dually based. Like other symptoms of social distress, it is deeply rooted in the sociological fabric. Unlike many such phenomena, however, it has a sharply defined medical aspect. It is to the difficulties and limitations of the medical aspect that we will now address ourselves.

8 Venereal Diseases as a Medical Problem

Apart from the regular and general medical examination of school-children, health promotion in this country has been largely programmed along the lines of prevention and detection of specific diseases. We take for granted, for example, repeated inspection by our dentist. Employer and employee alike accept as a matter of course the regular visits of a mass miniature radiography unit to their factory, and its role in helping to eradicate tuberculosis. Large-scale surveys to detect cases of diabetes have been a more recent development. The yearly clinical 'check-up' so common to the American scene, and the opportunity it affords for health education of the individual by the physician, has, however, little or no part in or out of our National Health Service. The value of general periodic medical examinations, in terms of allaying fears and improving prognosis, does have advocates in this country, and one hopes for more universal adoption. Meanwhile failure to see prevention in educational as well as clinical terms continues.

This is perhaps not surprising. As pointed out in *New Society* (20 December 1962), medical students receive their training almost exclusively in hospital, and are acquainted with rare conditions and exacerbations of familiar diseases. There is a need, it was stated, for wider teaching in regard to family background and preventive work. In our universities some medical faculty departments of Public Health, and Social and Preventive

Medicine have been more aware of these needs than others. Without inculcation of a sense of individual positive health by doctors, and its regular reinforcement, such specific educational and preventive programmes as we have are likely to remain limited in their value.

Public education in, and prevention of, venereal diseases has long been the statutory obligation of Local Health Authorities. The passing of the Health Services Act in 1946 made no difference to the role of the Medical Officer of Health in this respect. At the time of writing, however, very few Local Health Authorities are known to employ full-time non-medical and non-nursing Health Education Officers to carry out these tasks. One of these I know personally, and his aims in regard to venereal disease stem from a wide basis of health education. Questions of sex and its associated diseases branch naturally out of matters of personal hygiene. Courses of lectures, demonstrations, film strips and discussion groups at schools, youth clubs and welfare centres are aimed at giving the young factual knowledge, with a sense of citizenship and a consciousness of the needs for individual responsibility. The sexual problems of the young are freely discussed. The facts of human reproduction and all it implies emotionally are frankly faced. Sexually transmitted diseases, their root causes, course, prevention and treatment are outlined. At the other end of the scale are those Local Authorities who do no more than place notices – all too readily defaced or removed – in public lavatories, to indicate where and when treatment may be obtained. Such interpretation of statutory obligations leaves much to be desired.

Another agency which has taken part in public education, with hopes of prevention, is the Central Council for Health Education. It is financed by a voluntary levy on Local Authorities. From 1942 there was close collaboration between this body and the Ministry of Health, and large sums were spent during the last war. With the post-war fall in the incidence of venereal infections efforts declined. Whether they are recovering with sufficient force and speed to meet the rising tide of infection is a matter for speculation. Efforts have certainly been made by way of a nation-wide distribution of posters. These, however, have not always met with public acceptance. Short, well-written, factual accounts of venereal diseases, stressing the need for early treatment, have been made available for distribution through health and welfare departments and hospital clinics. The Central Council for Health Education has been increasingly active too in alerting Press, radio and television services to the facts of the present position. While the presentations which resulted were of varied quality, on the whole their educational value and impact have served long-term aims and helped to bring the facts of the situation today before the public.

In 1951 a new non-governmental agency was formed in this country. This is the British Federation against the Venereal Diseases. One of its aims is 'to encourage the spread of knowledge of the facts about venereal disease'. This body encompasses social as well as medical background and collaborates with others, nationally and internationally. Its chief links in this last respect are with the highly active International Union against the Venereal Diseases and Treponematoses, and with the Venereal Diseases and Treponematosis Division of the World Health Organization, centred in Geneva.

Few figures are available to measure the value of these and other efforts. In 1958[81] the British Federation against the Venereal Diseases reported its findings following interviews, by a trained and experienced social worker, of 292 patients attending a department of venereology in London. Two hundred and thirty-one of the patients were males and 61 were females. Only 73 had received any formal sex education as adolescents. Ten had seen leaflets concerning venereal disease. In 1963 Dr C. E. Gurr[38] of the Middlesex County Council sent questionnaires to 123 schools inquiring about sex education of girls. He received 115 replies. Eighty-four schools claimed to give sex teaching, through biology, science, personal hygiene, domestic science, physical and religious education and mothercraft, in the fourth year of senior schooling. In one area, health visitors and a doctor took part in talks with school-leavers. Fourteen schools

availed themselves of the services of Marriage Guidance
Counsellors and 49 employed films and film strips.

The latest information comes from Schofield's study on behalf
of the Central Council for Health Education and reported in
The Sexual Behaviour of Young People.[95] Schofield found that
16 per cent of boys and 13 per cent of girls aged 15–19 had no
knowledge of venereal diseases. Over half of the young people in
the study did not know anything of the signs and symptoms of
syphilis or gonorrhoea. A third were found to have learned
about venereal diseases from friends. Television and books
provided a further third with such information. Among other
sources were parents, schools and posters. Books and friends
proved the most accurate sources. Television tended to leave
people with only vague ideas about signs and symptoms.
Schofield concluded that although most young people have now
heard about venereal diseases there is still a good deal of
ignorance about the presenting signs and symptoms.

Sex education, an essential basis to factual knowledge about
venereal diseases, is itself a vexed question. The churches as a
whole see such education related specifically to moral and
Christian principles. What Christ called 'the good within' they
see as a natural endowment, apportioned, unlike intelligence or
wealth, in equal measure to all. The Christian teaching seeks to
nurture this talent. Other teachers of other religions place the
emphasis on other aspects. Mohammedanism teaches the
dangers of alcohol and warns that women lack moral sense.
Some see sex education as best taught from a basis of citizenship
and recommend discussion groups in community and welfare
centres. In general they recommend social orientation of both
parents and young, the health questions being dealt with by
doctors, health visitors and health educators. Yet others see the
problem as one for the home, the parents and the family circle,
answers being given as questions and problems arise. The
diffidence of many fathers and mothers, and their children, in
discussing sexual matters makes this a less obvious approach.
Undoubtedly there is more than enough scope for all approaches.

It is, however, right to caution that possession of facts or principles does not necessarily offer an impregnable bulwark against a flood of sexual emotion.

Any discussion of prevention would be incomplete without mention of prophylactic treatment. Simple expedients such as urinating and using soap and water as soon after exposure as possible, while no guarantee of protection, are generally recommended on the grounds of common sense and simple hygiene. It is perhaps worth reflecting on the war-time findings of Campbell.[13] According to these the incidence of infection among 277,000 brothel clients who used simple ablution and application of local prophylactics was only 31 per 100,000 over a period of eight months. It is not known for how long individual men were under observation.

It continues to be a bewildering paradox to many that, with condoms (French letters or sheaths) so readily and cheaply available, sexually transmitted diseases should be increasing. It is true that the original intention of the condom, when it was first introduced in the eighteenth century, was to minimize the chances of infection. Today it does no more than this. It is no guarantee against contaminated fingers. While the regular use of condoms by all promiscuous men and insistence on their use by their partners would reduce the number of infections among them, it is the experience of venereologists that condoms are very seldom used in casual exposures. They are more often used by the sophisticated and those practising regular intercourse with the same partner. A recent report from the Royal Navy's East Station shows the reasons given by 723 infected sailors, who failed to make use of the free issue of condoms.[20] The three main reasons were: carelessness, the influence of alcohol removing learnt restraints or rendering the man physically incapable of using the condom, and, thirdly, a misplaced faith in the bacteriological 'cleanliness' of the woman concerned.

Where exposure to possible infection has taken place early reporting, followed by prompt treatment in those found infected, is the most thoroughly practical measure. Much of the war-time educational effort was directed to this end. It was made clear to servicemen and women and civilians, through posters and newspaper articles and radio, that any risk of infection from irregular sexual behaviour should prompt medical examination at an early date. Worrying symptoms of any kind demanded immediate consultation. With his relish for the succinct phrase Tommy Atkins summed up this advice as 'better safe than sorry', and while it was often wished that he had taken the matter to heart at an earlier stage, the dictum served him and others well. The sick or worried man or woman all too readily gives way to rationalization, and the Tommy Atkins approach and preaching has been invaluable in creating a conditioned reflex. The principle of early reporting and prompt treatment is aimed not only at care and cure of the immediate patient but, through him, his sex partner, and the protection of the public health in general. Prompt treatment assures a high degree of disability limitations.

This is known only from the facts of follow-up examinations which are essential to the assurance of the future health of the patient. Modern treatment is usually straightforward and sometimes simple, but it is the repeated tests thereafter which guard the patient against the dangers of relapse, complications and subsequent disability. It is not always easy to bring an appreciation of these points to the patient who is so quickly relieved by modern therapy of a urethral or vaginal discharge, a rash or the abdominal pain of salpingitis. Even those initially found to be free from infection tend to ignore the fact that the maximum incubation period of syphilis is three months, and that they should therefore secure for themselves a final blood test at that time.

Apart from those who find themselves obviously in trouble and are finally diagnosed as having a venereal or other sexually transmitted disease or some other condition, many attend in a symptom-free state. Those who follow the 'better safe than sorry' dictum need not fear that the doctor will upbraid them for wasting his time. Venereologists view the care of such patients as an important and integral part of their preventive work and a welcome opportunity, not only to reassure the patient of his freedom from infection, but to impart factual information and to clear up doubts. The earlier this is done the better. Learning is easiest when those to be taught are at their most receptive. All too often men and women appear who for long have carried a burden of guilt about possible infection to the detriment of their health and well-being. Deeply rooted and unallayed fears have been known to deter people from the normal activities of a full life. A steady stream of patients who have been promiscuous or once risked infection seek examination and blood testing. Some do this a few weeks or months before marriage. The Matrimonial Causes Act of 1937 lays down that a marriage may be declared null and void if one partner knows he or she was suffering from a communicable venereal disease at the time of the ceremony. It is necessary for the offended partner to be unaware of the infection at the time of marriage, to institute proceedings within a year of the wedding, and to cease intercourse from the time of discovery of the infection. Some believe that wise counsels prevail in other countries. In many states of America pre-marital, and even pre-employment, blood testing for syphilis is obligatory.

Most of the patients attending a hospital clinic in this country do so of their own accord, making full use of the facility of direct access to the hospital consultant service. Those who first seek the advice of their family doctor are frequently referred. The need for a scientifically based diagnosis is nowadays more often recognized, and so sought, by both patient and family physician. With this end in view, some will seek the attention of a consultant venereologist, practising privately. Alternatively, as provided by the Health Service, a domiciliary consultation may be sought. Other out-patient and in-patient services, ante-natal clinics and blood transfusion units also refer patients. All properly organized ante-natal services carry out a routine blood test for syphilis, together with blood grouping and iron content studies, on every pregnant woman and at each of her pregnancies. All donors providing blood for transfusion have a blood test for syphilis carried out on each sample donated. This is considered obligatory under the provisions of the Pharmaceutical Substances Act (1956). It offers a most useful way of having a blood test to those who are shy about asking their practitioner and are reluctant to attend a special clinic. Where results of tests are other than negative, investigation is essential. Not unnaturally unexpected findings cause alarm. Fortunately most of those concerned, when made aware of the possible consequences of non-treatment, come to view the discovery as something of a blessing in disguise. As is so often the case, the doctor's concern is for the patient's future rather than his or her past.

Enough has been said to suggest that treatment of the infected individual, although a doctor's prime concern, is by itself not considered adequate. As in the case of all communicable diseases, the public's health requires protection. That all attendance at a special clinic is voluntary and confidential, however, places the venereologist, as indeed it does any doctor, in a delicate position. He must steer a policy course which, while respecting the rights and freedoms of the patient immediately in his care, seeks to prevent disability in others. By all the means at his disposal he must try to curtail the spread of infection generally. The guiding principle in all this is a basic epidemiological one. For every infection found at least another is sought. This principle the venereologist applies to all venereal and sexually transmitted diseases.

The first line of approach in securing attendance and examination of sex contacts is through the original patient. This is by no means always easily managed. A man with gonorrhoea may have only the haziest recollection of the girl he picked up at a dance hall or in a public-house. His exposure may well have taken place in an aura of alcohol. He may well have a degree of amnesia for the experience, cradled in remorse. None the less every effort is made to secure a detailed description of his consort, and if possible her full name and address. Although this is all too often an unrewarding exercise, time spent by the venereologist or his social worker is never wasted if it acquaints patients with their social obligations and the need for their cooperation in public health measures. Where useful information is forthcoming from a patient, it is usual to advise him that a too direct approach to discussion of his infection with the woman concerned will meet with rebuff and protestations of freedom from symptoms. These will stem from feminine modesty and lack of evidence of any infection. It would be better for the man to take an oblique line in advising the woman of her need to attend. 'I have had treatment for venereal disease. We have had intercourse. You should attend before you have symptoms.' To this approach women show an amenable common sense and usually present themselves without undue delay for examination. Many men will bring the woman or women concerned.

For the convenience of all, the man is given a numbered 'contact slip' to give to the woman. It shows the place and session times of her local clinic (the diagnosis concerned is added in code). This she is asked to present when she attends. Thus her doctor can deal adequately by way of examination and investigation; documents can be cross-referenced, and the highest degree of epidemiological control effected. Even where initial information is scanty and unpromising, men will sometimes undertake their own detective work and bring the consort or provide more adequate data at a later visit.

How efficient is the 'contact slip' in contact tracing? In 1954 Haworth and Nicol,[44] working in London, stated that the contact slip was most successful in cases where a wife or regular consort was involved. There was, however, a high failure rate among the hard core of cases where the man's exposure was with a casual contact. In 1963 Dunlop,[24] also working in London, secured the attendance of 24 women contacts in a series of 100 consecutive cases of men with gonorrhoea. Six only of the women were 'reservoir' contacts, the remainder being 'secondary' contacts, that is, wives or regular girl-friends. 'Clearly,' says Dunlop, 'the contact slip is an inefficient method for tapping the reservoir of gonorrhoea, and reliance on this method is one of the main reasons for failure of control of the disease.'

In some instances full details by way of name, address, age and description of the female are available, but the man, from disgust at his own behaviour or from disillusionment, may prefer to have no part in arranging for her attendance. In others the man may have done his best but failed to gain the woman's cooperation.

Besides the 'contact slip' two other regular methods are available to the venereologist. In these the original patient's name is not divulged unless he gives permission. These two methods may also be applied where speed seems to be a paramount consideration; for example, where the woman concerned is a prostitute or thought to be one of the many young women who roam the country and behave promiscuously. The first method is to write to the woman immediately, advising her that she has been named as being in contact with a serious infectious disease, and giving her an appointment to attend at an early date and if possible before symptoms appear. This method is particularly useful where she lives other than locally. In such a case she can be acquainted with the place and session times of special clinics in her own area. These are published in booklet form at regular intervals by the Ministry of Health and supplied to all clinics. As an alternative she may be advised to take the letter to her general practitioner.

Alternatively, or in addition, the venereologist may employ the second method. He may arrange through a Medical Officer of Health for the girl or woman to be visited by a specially trained health visitor, the position explained, her cooperation sought and attendance arranged. This is delicate work and requires a great deal of tact and experience. The natural disinclination of girls and women to believe that they are the victims of infection; modesty; fecklessness or resentment may require to be overcome. Willing help in this work is often forthcoming from general practitioners, ante-natal clinics, probation officers and school medical officers. Where the woman lives other than locally, or moves on to another town, her local Medical Officer of Health is alerted to the belief that he has a person with infectious disease in his area. He is asked to

arrange for her attendance. The local consultant venereologist
will be asked to look out for her and to make her welcome.
Following recent suggestions from venereologists that there is a
need for greater speed and more thorough cooperation in
contact tracing, the Ministry of Health is at present reviewing
methodology with a view to improving the 'yield' of contacts
and so effecting a greater degree of control.

Several stumbling-blocks require to be overcome. Firstly,
there is little information that contact tracing really effects
epidemiological control nationally or locally. Only one study[67]
seems to suggest that where all methods were employed the
percentage of gonococcal infections acquired in the area
covered was steadily reduced over a number of years. The area
was a county borough of some 141,000 population only.
Whether such methods, zealously and relentlessly pursued,
would work in larger cities, where the diseases are most concentrated, is unknown. The absence of such data no doubt
leads to pessimism and perhaps cynicism about the role and
value of contact tracing. Another difficulty is that health visitors,
who usually undertake the work, are employed by Local
Authorities and have no jurisdiction outside their own boun-
daries – indeed these are often jealously guarded. This may well
mean the difference between success and failure in securing the
attendance of a contact, for speed in the work is essential. Not
least of the difficulties is the individual doctor's views on freedom
of the citizen. He may also feel that he is on dangerous ground
legally. Even a paragraph in his contract, to the effect that his
'duties include any necessary action at his discretion for the
follow-up of any person suspected of suffering from a venereal
disease', may be so lacking in specificity as to make him wary.

If orientating patients and their casual sex contacts to an
appreciation of the consequences and implications of their
condition appears to be just routine work, much more is required where a spouse is involved. The more usual presentation
of this type of situation involves a man who has had marital
intercourse subsequent to an extra-marital exposure, and before
symptoms of disease are obvious. If the diagnosis is syphilis or

gonorrhoea his plight is a pitiable one. The confidential nature of care is as always scrupulously observed in such instances. A man's diagnosis is not revealed to his wife without his permission and, of course, vice versa. If the innocent spouse insists on knowing her own diagnosis he or she is told. The only reason for breach of confidence arises in court cases. Venereal infection may be overt evidence of infidelity and, as such, ground for divorce. The venereologist who is subpoenaed to give evidence in such cases must seek the protection of the Court if asked to reveal what has been imparted to him in the privacy of the consulting room. He cannot refuse to divulge information without committing contempt. Few cases do in fact end in the divorce court. Although wives are not credited with forgetfulness, they are generally forgiving; if not always thought to be practical they are certainly pragmatic and readily weigh the pros and cons of their position. The protection and cohesion of the marriage is very much in the forefront. If the marriage is basically a good one the man's misery will be matched only by the severely wounded pride of his wife. Experience shows that such a marriage will, with the aid of time, recover much of its earlier harmony. At the other extreme, in a poor or unstable partnership, the introduction of venereal infection may precipitate separation or divorce. Between these extremes lie those marriages where an infection may signal 'caution' and where the couple, tending to drift apart, are suddenly brought to a realization of what is really happening to them.

The role of contact tracing is shown here by two illustrative instances.

CASE 1. Mr A. B., a lorry driver in his twenties, was referred for consultation by his family doctor. The complaint was of urethral discharge of one day's duration. Extra-marital intercourse was admitted with a girl to whom he had offered a lift in his lorry six days previously. Marital intercourse had taken place two days before symptoms appeared. A diagnosis of gonorrhoea was established, its implications made clear and the patient's cooperation sought. Thirty-six hours later Miss C. D. attended. She stated that she had had a slight increase in vaginal discharge for two weeks but had not thought it remarkable, admitted intercourse with A. B. 8 days before and with another man two months previously. She was found to have gonorrhoea and treated. Although most willing to help in securing her earlier consort's attendance, she was unable to give more than his name. His home town was 150 miles distant. He had been visiting friends locally when she met him at a party, and she did not know his address. In the meantime Mr A. B., deeply miserable and contrite, felt enough confidence in his four-year-old marriage to tell his wife the full facts. She attended four days after her husband's initial visit. She denied intercourse with anyone other than her husband. A diagnosis of gonorrhoea was established and treatment given.

This case illustrates a straightforward piece of contact tracing with cooperative people, but shows how limited may be the tracing of the chain of infection. This is so on many occasions.

CASE 2. Between 11 October and 21 November, three men attended and were found to have early infectious syphilis. The descriptions of their source of infection were markedly similar. She was about 16 or 17 years old, short, thin and blonde. One man named her as Clarissa and believed she lived locally.

On 5 December a Miss H. S. attended and was found to have primary syphilis. She named two men, both of whom attended. One was her regular consort. He showed no evidence of infection up to two months from the time of his first attendance. The second man named did have syphilis. He believed his source of infection was a Miss Clarissa S., a sister of Miss H. S. Clarissa attended after a good deal of persuasion by her sister, the health visitor, a doctor's letter and the man who had named her. Widespread infectious syphilis was found. Sixteen days later a fifth man with syphilis also named Clarissa. He pointed out that she had dyed her hair black and had a missing left upper canine tooth, a feature noted by one of the original three men.

Two other cases of syphilis were traced from one of the original three. The fifth man was instrumental in securing the attendance of another woman. After nine weeks of regular examinations, when she defaulted, there was no evidence of infection.

This case illustrates the difficulties of tracing where descriptions are meagre. The part that may be played by one highly infectious and promiscuous woman in effecting an outbreak must be obvious.

What of the discovery of a long-standing congenital or acquired syphilis which has been non-infectious for many years? Such cases are referred from other hospital departments, ante-natal clinics and blood transfusion centres. Once diagnosis is fully established and treatment commenced, the need to examine other members of the patient's family is clear. Like-wise, in the case of a woman in her early forties, found to have neuro-syphilis, there is an indication to examine the husband. That he has no symptoms augurs well for him. It is certainly, in the circumstances, the best time to see him. If he is found to have syphilis in latent form he, and his family, may be assured that treatment will protect him from late crippling or killing compli-cations. Children of the marriage will clearly need blood testing also. Similarly, in the case of the young expectant mother, found to be a congenital syphilitic, there is need to alert her brothers and sisters as well as her parents to the necessity of early examination. In all these situations, which demand patience and sympathetic understanding by everyone concerned, the aim is prevention of potential tragedy and all the varied and domestic problems which can arise from chronic illness and the prema-ture loss of a parent.

In the U.S.A. much has recently been made of a method of finding patients known as 'cluster testing'. This consists of seeking the attendance of men and women moving in a social milieu in which the organisms of venereal disease are known to be circulating. The technique will be recognized as an extension of contact-tracing as just described. 'Cluster testing' is part of the programme of the United States task force, set up in 1961 with the avowed aim of eradicating syphilis in that country by 1972. The total effort includes twice-yearly visits by health visitors to all doctors, to gain cooperation in learning about syphilitics and their sexual and social contacts. Personal inter-views with these are sought, as indeed they are with all syphi-litics, whether treated privately or at public clinics.

The tracing is vigorously and relentlessly pursued, and every pressure is put on the people concerned to seek examina-tion. The need for the individual concerned to show a fit sense of social responsibility to his fellows is freely used in the coercion. Those employed on the task are university graduates, many with degrees in social studies. All are specially trained in the psychology of persuasion and apply it with a dedication which is said to be remarkable. Public education and close scrutiny and surveillance of some 8,000 laboratories carrying out blood tests for syphilis are included in the task.

The U.S. Public Health Service reported in 1962[104] that, starting from a basis of 5,452 patients with early infectious syphilis, they were able to bring to treatment, by ordinary methods of contact tracing, 2,047 other persons. By interview and examination of 'cluster suspects' another 487 infected people were found.

There is no report of 'cluster testing' in this or any other country. Indeed there must be some doubt as to whether the British temperament would acquiesce in such revolutionary and high-powered methods of persuasion of social as well as sexual contacts of syphilis. However, it must be made clear that specific efforts are made here to examine high percentages of recognizably 'at risk' groups as a matter of routine. This applies, for example, to men and women prisoners. From 1951 to 1956 Elizabeth Keighley[52] working at H.M. Prison at Holloway, London, found that 16·7 per cent of all women prisoners had syphilis or gonorrhoea. Furthermore, under the Criminal Justices Act (1948) magistrates, now more frequently than ever before, remand women on charges of prostitution for a medical report. Young girls on remand who are known to have had intercourse, and unmarried mothers-to-be, are regularly referred. Statutory tests are required for girls who absent themselves without leave from approved schools. In some areas probation officers and socially orientated policewomen advise the attendance for tests of girls and young women found missing from home and known to have been living with promiscuous men. All these efforts are particularly useful not only to the unsuspecting sufferers but because they provide a method of tapping the reservoir of undiagnosed, asymptomatic female disease.

*

Something of the problems of clinical and laboratory diagnosis in all forms of sexually transmitted diseases has already been mentioned in the section relevant to the various conditions. Improvements in laboratory techniques have been effected in the last quarter-century in regard to the less common conditions. More recently detection of the trichomonas vaginalis by culture methods has been greatly improved. The discovery that the transport or travelling medium used for the gonococcus will also maintain the parasite in a viable state for a few days has been of great assistance. If research currently being undertaken confirms the belief of many that non-specific urethritis is a virus disease, then the way will be opened for much more direct and definite diagnosis and for better understanding of the epidemiology of this increasingly common condition.

In gonorrhoea the essential problems of diagnosis are many. Apart from the fact that there are difficulties in persuading women to attend for examination, accurate and prompt diagnosis at the first testing is, at present, not always possible. Such failure is all too readily seized upon by women to excuse themselves further attendance, and so for some 20 per cent the first attendance is the last. Such tests as we have are by no means infallible. Repeated testing is essential.

The laboratory side of this problem is currently being tackled along two main lines. Standard culture methods are under review and recently a medium has been developed whose fundamental nutritional ingredients ensure selective growth of the gonococcus, with suppression of growth of all other organisms which might be present. The yield of isolations of gonococci in named contacts and others is being increased, it is claimed. While this is improvement, it is still far from offering anything like 'instant' diagnosis to all those infected.

The second approach to the problem is by a technique found successful in locating other bacteria. This is the method known as fluorescent antibody testing. It depends on the fact that certain dyes fluoresce or appear illuminated when seen in ultra-violet light. Some of these dyes are capable of effecting a biochemical union with the type of proteins which develop and circulate as antibodies in the body of an infected host. Such anti-bodies, prepared in living animals, when conjugated with fluorescent dye component, are still capable of attacking organisms, and these in turn therefore show up, in a micro-scope illuminated with an ultra-violet light lamp, as greenish-yellow fluorescences. This direct method of detecting gonococci in smears has so far proved unsuitable for instant diagnosis. The so-called delayed method, however, is diagnostically quicker at twenty-four hours than the standard culture methods requiring two to five days. An indirect fluorescent test-ing method, whereby an attempt is made to detect gonococcal antibodies in the prospective patient's blood by use of a test organism, is also under investigation. It suffers from the deficiency of other blood tests for gonorrhoea in that not all sufferers from the disease show circulating antibodies, and in some the development of those may be minimal and delayed. The development of a reliable serological test – a blood test – for the early diagnosis of gonorrhoea is an urgent require-ment. Such a test would be useful for the identification of carriers, especially those females who form the reservoir of infection.

Problems of laboratory diagnosis of syphilis have in the recent past been concentrated on blood tests. In the whole field of venereology nothing has called forth so much expenditure of time and effort as the attempt to find a reliably diagnostic test for this disease. Though the T.P.I. test is near perfection, it is a highly complicated, lengthy and not inexpensive procedure. The search therefore continues. In the meantime, reliance for diag-nosis is often placed on a battery of tests on repeated specimens of the patient's blood.

Currently under investigation, and of some promise, is the fluorescent treponemal antibody test (F.T.A.). The technique used is the indirect method, in which dead treponemes are used to detect antibodies in the prospective patient's blood. The test is certainly specific and only a little more liable to give false results than the T.P.I. test. It is, relatively, a straightforward, quick and inexpensive test. For all these reasons it has a much greater chance of adoption for routine purposes than many of its competitors.

Another problem of syphilis diagnosis is the occasional need for speed in certain circumstances. Rapid but highly sensitive methods have been used. For example, where large numbers of Mexicans seek to enter the Southern States of the United States at harvest time such rapid tests, often performed with a few drops of blood on a card or a tile, prove most suitable. Those found with positive blood reactions require more detailed investigation with standard procedures.

The treatment of all the sexually transmitted diseases has been much improved in the last twenty-five years. The most recent addition to the therapeutic armament has been metronidazole for trichomonal infestation, most of the attendant problems of which have been mentioned. While there is no evidence from animal experiments or human medication of danger to the foetus, it is generally agreed to be a wise policy to avoid giving the drug, like so many others, during the early months of pregnancy. There is nothing so far to suggest that the trichomonas is becoming resistant to metronidazole, and this drug looks like having a long and useful life.

In the absence of a recognized cause of non-specific urethritis, treatment of the condition remains empirical. Whether full understanding of the cause would solve the problem of therapy is doubtful. Not all virus diseases, especially those with a natural tendency to relapse and recurrence, are readily amenable to such antibiotics as are at present available. Cure rates are fairly good, although cure is unpredictable in the individual patient. Furthermore, we are still far from being able to forecast with confidence that any form of treatment will be helpful in those with complications.

The advent of penicillin in 1943 effected a revolution in the treatment of both syphilis and gonorrhoea. Prolonged and hazardous therapy for syphilis and the waning success of the sulphonamides in gonorrhoea were replaced almost overnight by short, safe and curative courses of treatment. Well-designed trials of penicillin soon determined minimal dosage schedules, especially for syphilis. Time has proved these effective, and with minor variations they have been accepted throughout the world.

In the more prolonged courses of penicillin used for syphilis the patient may develop sensitivity to the drug by way of an itchy rash or general reaction. Occasionally more serious reactions have taken place, and in America sudden deaths from the shock of a high degree of sensitivity have been reported. So far there is no satisfactory test to determine who is and who is not sensitive to penicillin. This is a great pity because, being in such regular use, it is the cause of nearly half of all the sensitivities seen in skin departments. In the event of an individual patient being sensitive to penicillin, biologically active equivalent doses of another antibiotic, such as one of the tetracycline group, are prescribed.

Recently Collart and his colleagues in Paris[19] have made some effort to determine why the T.P.I. test alone should remain positive in a high percentage of adequately treated syphilitics. Repetitive and laborious work with glands from rabbits and humans showed the presence, by staining methods, of what those workers believed to be treponema pallidum, in those fully and adequately treated and followed up. In both rabbits and humans treatment was delayed. Of ten human patients all but one had had repeated courses of penicillin over one to sixteen years. The organisms found appeared to preserve vitality but not virulence. There was some evidence that the state of equilibrium between host and treponeme, which we call cure, may be upset by factors which are as yet little understood. There is of course need for confirmation of these findings, need for identification of the organism as that of human syphilis, and need to eliminate the possibility of re-infection, before the implications regarding our concepts of clinical cure can be seriously challenged. Even then, many must doubt that our present ideas about cure can be shaken.

Regular consorts of infectious syphilitics, it has been pointed out, are particularly liable to develop syphilis. For this reason, and more especially in America, 'abortive' treatment is frequently given in such cases. This would be exceptional practice in this country,[116] where the principle of diagnosis before treatment is highly regarded. The following case illustrates some typical difficulties.

Mr S. H., a homosexual railway clerk of 29, was found to have secondary syphilis. He had many lesions in his mouth which were highly infectious and which had been present for some weeks. Ten days prior to his attendance, Mr S. H. had made the first of three visits to his dentist, who had carried out fillings and a scraping.

Contact was made with the dentist concerned, warning him that he should consider the situation and perhaps attend for examination and discussion. The alternatives open to him were twofold. Either he should be on the sick list for three months with repeated examinations and tests, avoiding meanwhile both work and sex, or he should have a course of 'abortive' penicillin. He chose the second and was advised therefore that he should submit to follow-up for the two years of tests recommended for everyone treated for early syphilis.

In gonorrhoea the aim of therapy has been to effect a 100 per cent cure rate with a single injection of penicillin. In the 1940s and early 1950s cure rates of 95 per cent and more were achieved in large series of cases without difficulty. Since about 1956 it has been the experience of workers in many parts of the world that failure to respond, or a relapse, has been more common than ever before, even to dosage rates four to eight times as great as those effective little over a decade ago. A spiral of increasing failure rates alternating with increasing penicillin dosage schedules has begun. In cases of repeated failure very large or multiple doses, daily or bi-daily over several days, are now not uncommon. No gonococcus completely resistant to penicillin has yet been described though there is clear laboratory evidence in this country and elsewhere[21, 118] that strains or varieties of the responsible organism have emerged which are less sensitive than others and less sensitive too than their ancestors. Such strains are sometimes described as partially resistant. Whether this is the direct result of low dosage in past years, or a mutation of the gonococcus, has not been settled. The situation is confused by conflicting theories. The mode of action of penicillin is not clearly understood. It seems possible that low levels of penicillin in the patient's blood, while insufficient to kill gonococci, may have prompted the organism to adopt internal bio-chemical changes which enable it to adapt satisfactorily to a penicillin environment. This happened to the gonococcus in the sulphonamide era. Within a few years from its inception the drug was quite useless in 75 per cent of all gonorrhoeal infections. A second possibility is that too low a standard dosage of penicillin in past years may have aided the survival and selective spread of the less sensitive strains, so that their percentage of the present-day gonococcal population has increased to a noticeable degree. Mutation, the other suggested reason, implies a spontaneous and usually unpredictable internal change in bio-chemical construction. Such a possibility cannot be excluded at this time.

A further difficulty is the emergence of what is known as cross-resistance, i.e. some degree of resistance to more than one antibiotic may exist. In the case of streptomycin, an antibiotic also commonly used as routine injection treatment of gonorrhoea, especially in France, a strain of gonococci completely resistant to it has been found. Nearly half the gonococcal strains which are partially resistant to penicillin are wholly resistant to streptomycin. Similar phenomena are expected to become commoner.

Such drugs as penicillin and streptomycin have the great advantage of being suitable for 'one-shot', curative, intra-muscular dosage at the time of diagnosis. (They have the added advantage of being cheap.) Thus the venereologist can feel happy on two counts. Firstly, a treated patient leaving his department stands a high chance of being non-infectious within, at most, twenty-four hours. Secondly, and as a corollary, the public health is safeguarded. Where, because of an individual's sensitivity to penicillin, other antibiotics have to be prescribed, these points are less easily met. The 'strategic reserve' of antibiotics, particularly the tetracyclines and new penicillins, are not generally suitable for intra-muscular injection. They have to be taken by mouth at regular intervals, by day and night for several days. Patients are forgetful. The need for a regular routine may give rise to awkward questions at home. In avoiding these, there may be a break-down of the essential régime. Venereologists do not, as a rule, fail to remind the pharmaceutical houses at every opportunity of the anxiety about the future role of penicillin in gonorrhoea. So far these firms have not responded with an adequate substitute with all the ideal qualities of penicillin in its first decade. It may well be that some of the new penicillins, at present of limited value in gonorrhoea, can be prepared to give high and active blood levels over twenty-four to forty-eight hours after injection. Early attention to such matters seems important if gonorrhoea is not to become an expensive disease.

In the United States of America an attempt has been made to achieve what Carpenter[15] called 'antibiotic quarantine' in female patients with gonorrhoea. This was done by Hookings and Graves,[45] who gave not only curative doses of penicillin, but additional doses (at the same time) of a long-acting type of penicillin with a view to preventing re-infection of those patients during the ensuing fortnight. It was envisaged that this would not only give time for contact tracing, but would diminish the reservoir of infection. They claimed good results for their area over a two-year period. A similar attempt in Manchester[67] conducted over a year or more was associated with a rising incidence of disease in both males and females.

This takes us to a consideration of what has become known as 'epidemiological treatment' in gonorrhoea.[116] Where, for example, there is sound epidemiological information that a female is probably infected with gonorrhoea but immediate microscopic examination of specimens taken at her first attendance are negative, some venereologists offer treatment.

Mr A. C. reported on a Thursday that he had a urethral discharge of four days' duration. He was found to have acute urethral gonorrhoea. He admitted intercourse with two young women seven and five days previously. The earlier consort reported on Friday and was found to be infected. The later consort was known to be promiscuous. She had attended erratically when infected the previous year. She was located by a health visitor and invited to attend. She did so on

Saturday. Gonococci were not found in stained 'smear' preparations. The probability of infection and the limitation of 'instant' diagnostic methods was explained. Epidemiological treatment was offered and accepted.

Some venereologists hold to the principle that treatment before diagnosis is one from which there should rarely be any departure.[57] Considerations on behalf of the individual are prime and paramount. She is asked to share the burden of the responsibility for the public health, which is seen as secondary. In contrast, the first school of thought puts the emphasis on the public health aspect, recognizing the difficulties of persuading many women to attend, the problems of diagnosis and the possibility of an immediate (20 per cent) default. Epidemiological treatment is favoured by some venereologists as especially applicable to the prostitute and the young promiscuous female who admits to being the possible or probable source of a man's disease. In the case of secondary contacts, such as wives or regular girl-friends who are willing and wise enough to attend for repeated examination, the question of epidemiological treatment is less often applicable. In the case of the married woman legal considerations have to be taken into account.

It must be stated that there is no statistical or other demographic proof that epidemiological treatment helps to halt rising rates of incidence of gonorrhoea, and none would dissent from the Ministry of Health report for as long ago as 1958[90] that penicillin 'had made no lasting improvement in the incidence of gonorrhoea'. Venereologists in large centres of population are however conscious of a growing number of asymptomatic but possibly infectious women who leave their departments, probably for ever, to swell the reservoir of undiagnosed infection. It remains to be seen therefore whether the rising levels of gonorrhoea will dictate a new balance between clinical and epidemiological considerations.

Homosexual men with rectal infections receive treatment similar to others. Occasionally they prove difficult to cure and repeated courses of treatment may be required. The explanation for these failures is, at present, partly theoretical. It is thought that organisms producing an antidote called penicillinase may be present in the bowel, and thus the action of the antibiotic may be inhibited.

Robert Lees, venereologist at Edinburgh, is reputed to have said some years ago 'Any fool can treat a gonorrhoea but it takes an expert to define cure'. Even if the first half of this aphorism is not so clear-cut nowadays, the second can be held to be sounder than ever. Not unnaturally, patients tend to be interested in their own recovery. Each therefore should know that cure may be apparent rather than real and take care to have repeated tests after treatment. Patterns of follow-up vary little in this country. Generally patients are advised to report three times within the first week or two of treatment, for examinations and tests, and thereafter at longer intervals, with a final check at the end of three months. Following treatment for syphilis, examinations and blood tests are indicated at monthly intervals for six months, and thereafter three-monthly up to some two years at least. No matter how thoroughly the patient attends for treatment, relapse, with or without symptoms and signs, is always a possibility. Regular attendance will not only lead to detection of this but will find it at its most readily curable.

No less in other conditions, the necessity to ensure that the patient is cured of his or her infection is a problem which the doctor views most seriously. He knows that the absence of symptoms is the poorest of criteria and that only repeated tests can give assurance of cure. That the patient does not share this view, and takes much for granted, shows a serious need for public education in this respect. In some patients default from treatment and surveillance is perhaps understandable. Re-attending the clinic revives old guilt feelings which they find hard to bear. Many have to be nursed through these difficulties until cured. Much may be at stake for the patient and the family.

The need in surveillance is not only to ensure that the original infection has been cured but also that the patient is not incubating syphilis. One reason for aiming at the smallest possible dose of penicillin compatible with cure in gonorrhoea has been the fear of masking a concomitantly acquired and incubating syphilis. Time has shown this to be an exaggerated fear. Nevertheless it continues to be customary to advise patients to have a final blood test for syphilis three months after treatment of gonorrhoea. What the consensus of opinion on this point will be when the standard dosage of penicillin in gonorrhoea reaches levels recognized as known to abort incubating syphilis, remains to be seen.

In smaller departments, especially in the provinces, where a high percentage of the patients are local inhabitants, follow-up examinations are more readily completed. In larger towns and in the cities where the venereal diseases are concentrated, default is the rule rather than the exception, because of the greater mobility of city peoples, especially the young. There are men and women who seem to be constantly on the move in search of new work, on leave from the services, or between trips as merchant seamen. Long-distance lorry drivers, tourists and travellers on business are also recognized as being 'at risk'. Special provision is made for such patients through the aid of a standard travelling card (Ministry Form VI5). This little booklet is initiated by the clinic making the diagnosis. It gives the patient's clinical and laboratory findings, treatment and the results of follow-up tests. Diagnosis is in code. Armed with this and the locale and times of clinics on the way of his proposed itinerary, the patient is advised to present himself for such treatment or examinations as may be required. Similar arrangements exist at international level.

When patients default from treatment or surveillance, most venereologists operate some form of 'case-holding' technique. Routine or personal letters and, if necessary, visits by a trained health visitor to the home or place of work are arranged. Letters are usually placed in two sealed envelopes, the inner being non-commitally addressed for return to sender, and the outer clearly marked for personal attention only. The problem of visiting defaulters is likewise undertaken with thought and tact. The patient's needs are the first consideration in these matters.

The whole problem of case-holding bristles with doubts and difficulties. A report from Leeds in 1953[46] said that regular attendance, after default, in patients with gonorrhoea was rare, and that both men and women were quite impervious to personal or other influences in the matter. Others have believed that letters and visits to secure completion of surveillance are not unavailing and that whereas men respond more frequently to letters, women respond to personal visits. In the case of syphilis follow-up is vital, and this was underlined by a report in 1954.[74] Two hundred and sixty-eight men and women who had defaulted from syphilis treatment or surveillance during the decade 1941–50 were written to and, where necessary, visited; 183 (68 per cent) were located and 144 attended for reappraisal of their condition. According to the criteria defined, 51 required further surveillance and 32 required further treatment. Four of these were candidates for symptomatic neuro-syphilis. The great majority of those requiring to do so attended regularly after recall.

Although venereologists are at pains to prevent default it must be confessed that where the need is greatest – in large cities – their success, even with 'case-holding' techniques, is at its lowest.

The practice of venereology is securely based on an appreciation of the fundamental principles of chemistry, physics and biology. The elaboration of these principles in bio-chemistry, bacteriology and pharmacology, together with those of epidemiology and statistics, has placed at command a scientific approach to both diagnosis and treatment. The application of all this knowledge, more especially since the introduction of penicillin, guarantees clinical cure of gonorrhoea, syphilis, the less common venereal diseases and other sexually transmitted conditions, but it has made no lasting impression at the epidemiological level – indeed recrudescences threaten substantial gains. The death rate from congenital syphilis began to decline with the establishment of clinics and the introduction of new anti-syphilitic drugs. At that time some 1,200 infants died annually of the disease in England and Wales. At present, even one death a year is an extreme rarity. Likewise the incidence of congenital syphilis found in the 0–5 year age group has declined rapidly. Ministry of Health reports studied by the Office of Health Economics[100] show this improvement in terms of congenital syphilitic blindness. Whereas in the 1930s this cause accounted for approximately 12 per cent of all blindness, by 1960 the incidence had fallen to 0·46 per cent. In the case of acquired syphilis the gains are no less striking. From a death rate from the disease of 140 per million at the time the clinics were being opened, this had fallen to little over 10 per million by 1962. While acquired syphilis accounted for 6 per cent of blindness in the 1930s it contributed only a negligible percentage by 1960. Gonococcal infection of babies' eyes at the time of their delivery contributed one third of those children entering provincial schools for the blind in 1922. It was by far the greatest single cause. Now it is extremely rare. The rising gonorrhoea rate, however, calls for caution.

In the case of syphilis these gains are again threatened by the steadily rising incidence of early infection. Laird[64] has pointed out that the fall in the incidence of congenital syphilis is more readily accounted for by the fall in early syphilis than by any direct method used for prevention, such as ante-natal blood testing. No similar analysis is available to account for the falling incidence of late syphilis. The problem here is more complex. That an association does exist between the number of early infections and the incidence of late complications is, however, not doubted. The basic concept in these considerations is that not all early syphilis cases come forward for diagnosis and treatment; perhaps only four in five, or at best, nine in ten.

Gains by way of avoidance of crippling arthritis from gonorrhoea are less easily defined but are believed to be substantial. The situation is clearer with another complication. Gonorrhoea has in the past been a common source of sterility, especially in females. It has, until lately, been a less common cause of that condition. Now, as in syphilis, the present recrudescence of gonorrhoea threatens these gains. Guthe,[41] writing from the World Health Organization in Geneva, gave his opinion in 1958 as follows: 'The total reservoir of gonorrhoea does not appear to have been appreciably reduced in spite of the effectiveness of penicillin treatment in the individual'. By 1961[40] he was drawing attention, not only to the rising gonorrhoea rates in fifteen out of twenty-two countries studied, but also to the increasing frequency of complications. He quoted a report from Sweden which recorded that 10 per cent of women with gonorrhoea had the condition complicated by salpingitis, and 2–3 per cent of all cases were rendered sterile by their disease.

It must be admitted then that treatment – preventive or curative – as we have found it today is unlikely to control the spread of venereal and other sexually transmitted diseases. Now, as throughout their recorded history, their ubiquity makes them seem inevitable. If a defeatist attitude is not to be accepted there are two possible ways along which we may travel. Let us as a final analysis see whether either of these, the sociological or the medical, offers any hope for the control of venereal diseases tomorrow.

9   Variations on an Enigma

The particular phenomenon with which we are concerned is a world-wide one and the answer for us in Great Britain, if there is one, will necessarily differ from that of other societies with their own levels of development, religions and customs. Unwin's[105] study of the marriage mores and customs of some eighty primitive societies reveals that social development, discovery, expansion and other signs of an emerging and energetic society made their appearance only when rules and regulations were rigidly enforced. Societies with high-level incidences of pre-marital and extra-marital intercourse were lazy and unprogressive. These observations are germane in that they emphasize, even in a highly developed and sophisticated society such as ours, the need for conscious thought about where we wish to stand in the future in terms of sexual, as well as more general social, organization.

The most readily recognizable framework within which a society orders its affairs is its legal ordinances. The law is therefore another general factor which we must consider in looking to the future of venereal diseases. While it is not possible, as Lord Stoneham[91] recently pointed out, to make people moral by Act of Parliament, laws do have the general effect of setting standards and bounds to behaviour. It is pertinent therefore to ask if the law can offer anything for the future, particularly with some of the recognizable groups who are at special risk to infection.

The punitive legal measures of the last century and such

punishments as 'stoppages' of the proficiency pay of infected servicemen, which operated in the early part of this century, have proved of very little value in cutting incidence rates. Laws and regulations, similar to those originating in pre-war Sweden and developed with modifications in several countries, have not found favour here. These laws concerned notification of all cases of venereal disease and compulsory treatment. A British Mission studied them in 1937. Laird[68] advocated, but without success, that they be implemented in Britain. Decreasing prevalences of infection followed in those countries which adopted the laws, but similar decreases occurred in this country without them. There is no body of opinion in Britain in favour of their introduction now. The ending of the legalized control of brothels and prostitution in other countries has already been found to contribute little to the solution of the problem of controlling the spread of infection. The Street Offences Act, which was directed primarily at one of the root causes of infection, has had no more success.

Recent legal restrictions on the entry of immigrants into Britain have slowed down the rate of increase in the number of gonococcal infections. In 1964 the percentage contributed by male immigrants was the lowest for some years. The recent trend for West Indian women to join their menfolk here should be encouraged, since it is likely to promote stability in sexual relationships. An official policy of accepting families into the country (which applies to U.K. citizens going to Commonwealth countries) rather than itinerant unattached males or females is likely to be helpful. It would be welcomed as a declared aim of immigration policy.

The legal position of male homosexuals who contribute significantly to the total of venereal infections has been under review. The Wolfenden Report recommended that homosexual practices between consenting males in private should no longer be a crime. The subject was recently discussed in the House of Lords, which found in favour of the Wolfenden recommendation. Leave to introduce a Bill to this effect in the Commons was later refused. The Wolfenden Report said that there are realms of private behaviour which are outside the law. Lord Devlin, on the other hand, in his book *The Enforcement of Morals*,[23] states that there are areas of private behaviour where the law may require to interfere. He has in mind instances, some concerned with homosexuality, where the ordinary man considers that society is being offended. The burden of his thesis is that occasional coercion by the law in setting limits to private behaviour is more likely to bring about a healthy society. The crux of the situation would appear to be, therefore, whether the present social climate offers an auspicious time for implementing the Wolfenden recommendation. In the present atmosphere of 'permissiveness' it seems unlikely that discussion of a Bill in the Commons can be long delayed.

That public opinion already views homosexuality more liberally than ever before is reflected in the increasing readiness with which homosexual contact, as a source of disease, is admitted by patients. The number of homosexuals, now celibate, who would practice this type of sexual intercourse, or the degree of promiscuity among homosexuals, is unlikely to increase significantly with any new legislation. In our immediate context therefore it is doubtful whether the Bill at present before the Commons will, if passed, make any marked impact on venereal disease rates.

Removal of male homosexuality from the list of crimes would be welcomed by some venereologists. Fortunately the law treats the doctor's position as privileged, so the homosexual can be assured of thoroughly humane and confidential care.

This brings us to a consideration of private behaviour which is outside the law yet has anti-social traits. There are, for example, the increasing symptoms of social pathology in the behaviour of the girls and young women who, like homosexuals and immigrants, have already been identified as an 'at risk' group.

Here is an illustration:

Dorothy first attended the special clinic one afternoon on her way home from school. She was 15 years of age. She was found to have early syphilis, having been infected by a calling tradesman. It was not her first sexual experience. Dorothy attended daily, as advised, and was fully treated. Her parents were not informed. During the period of early post-treatment surveillance she defaulted. A month was allowed to pass, then another, without action. Thereafter a health visitor called at her home to make discreet inquiries. Dorothy had run away and had not been seen for six weeks or so. In due course she was found and returned to her family. Two months later she was known to be three months pregnant. A healthy, syphilis-free child was born and Dorothy elected to bring it up with the help of her mother.

Juvenile delinquency (with a sex ratio of ten males to one female) appears to be a male prerogative, but whether girls do, in fact, create so much less in the way of problems to society must be questioned. If it can be agreed that our standards and limits in matters of behaviour, delinquent *vis-à-vis* anti-social, are arbitrary, then we can re-appraise with minimal bias the activities of that minority of girls whose uninhibited conduct causes distress. The basis of the thesis is that while boys have in recent years increasingly offended against the written law, girls have been no less active in offending against the unwritten.

In support of this general contention can be cited the propensity of young girls, in revolt against parental control, to disappear from home without trace. Since no crime is committed, no figures are available. Those who deal with the problem – policewomen, children's officers and probation officers – report that the number of runaway girls is increasing to a disturbing extent. Over 100 runaway girls are currently being found annually by the police in a city of half a million. About half the girls are locals, the remainder usually from other towns and cities. Not infrequently they associate with promiscuous men, living with several in turn on a semi-permanent basis and using their sex as a passport to clothing, shelter, food and care. Running away from home is one way to promiscuity; for a minority it leads to outright prostitution, with venereal infection and illegitimate pregnancy as common consequences. It has already been noted that venereal infection has increased five times more in adolescent girls than in boys of the same age range and that two thirds of females with gonorrhoea are in the age group 15–24. The illegitimacy rate for England and Wales was 4·6 per cent of all births in 1955, rising steadily to 7·4 per cent (59,000) in 1963. Schofield[95] found that of the 17 per cent of girls aged 15–19 in his series who gave a history of pre-marital sexual intercourse, one in three became pregnant. Such figures are commonly quoted as indices of promiscuity. More important perhaps is the re-infection rate, which for gonorrhoea is as high as 10 per cent a year for females in some large cities.

Illegitimacy raises many problems apart from adoption, fostering and the growing number of unwanted children in Local Authority care. Among the most distressing, if distant, problems are those arising through the upbringing of children by proxy and without the presence of a father. Nurture in such circumstances gives poor prospects for maturity and sound citizenship. This is well recognized to be productive of 'misfits'.

There is also a growing tendency among girls to attempt suicide. As a clinical group attempted suicides are distinct from successful suicides. The age, sex, background and mentality of those involved is quite different in the two groups.[99] Attempted suicide is six to eight times more common than suicide and predominates in females, especially in those under 20.[84] The number of girls and young women under 20 with a diagnosis of attempted suicide is not accurately known, but it must be more than two and a half thousand per annum in England and Wales.

Running away from home, promiscuous behaviour, turning prostitute, illegitimate pregnancy and sometimes a suicide attempt may be associated in one and the same girl. All the phenomena are recognized as associated with all sexually trans-mitted disease; more frequently than not the girl is asympto-matic. The indications for relevant investigations are therefore more often social than medical. This observation calls for alert-ness amongst social workers and doctors and even parents with recalcitrant daughters, if control of the spread of infection is to be improved.

The growth of the phenomena described, even if at present marginal, is worth close attention. The most liberal interpretation of their behaviour is that the girls are mentally confused. They are searching, even appealing, for release from feelings of insecurity, isolation and a general meaninglessness in their lives. Their behaviour is characterized by attention-seeking and emotional vulnerability. A harsher but perhaps more objective view is that we are dealing with delinquency expressed in female terms.

The prevention of social breakdown devolves primarily on parents, but they need the support of society's structure. In the present state of affairs, which is likely to continue for some time, our best hope lies in earlier recognition of when a girl, and no less a boy, is in need of care and control. Distraught parents should be encouraged to seek prompt help, either formally or informally, in the hope that overt anti-social behaviour, and all that this may mean for the individual concerned and the family, will be forestalled. The recent Longford Committee report, which proposes dealing with such social problems through 'family courts', has some promise in this respect. A White Paper on this subject has recently been published. Re-organization of necessary work for the young is already under way in Scotland. Youth advisory services, similar to the one set up by Dr Faith Spicer in London, may also have a place in providing youth with guidance on social and sexual questions.

McElligott,[72] sometime adviser on venereal diseases to the Ministry of Health, summed up the situation thus: 'I cannot help feeling that if we took more trouble in looking after our growing girls, the reservoir of venereal disease could be reduced.'

Many patients both male and female do not of course show such extreme forms of aberrant behaviour. In many of them one or more of a great variety of personal influences and factors appear to dominate, as leading to venereal disease. For example, earnings higher than a young man can manage may lead to abuse of alcohol and so to infection. Conflict in the home and declarations of independence can be more readily supported by a young adult commanding a regular and high income. Thus an increasing proportion of young people now live in flats apart from their parents. Opportunities for sexual intercourse are thereby increased. In married men infection may follow seeking solace with another woman after a marital tiff or when a wife is pregnant and uninterested in sexual intercourse.

For some young people the home background appears to offer little support. Fully employed mothers and absence of active leadership in family affairs by fathers deprive young people of a pattern of well-ordered domestic arrangements, modes of behaviour, use of leisure and the need for foresight, which are worthy of imitation and necessary for satisfactory development. Young adults growing and living in homes replete with 'everything' may be denied interest in their hopes and aspirations. Many are left to their own devices in the evenings and at week-ends and are thus provided with opportunities for sexual intercourse. Unchaperoned teenage parties do likewise. Schofield[95] has shown that the home of one or other parent is the location of the first sexual intercourse in a high proportion of the 15- to 19-year-olds. He found this to be so for 50 per cent of boys and 43 per cent of girls admitting full sexual experience.

Such findings should alert parents to a sense of caution.

Complications will inevitably come to some families. For the majority of parents, however, hazarding the potential good name and happiness of their offspring by giving too much liberty too early has no place in their ideas of an adequate upbringing. This practice is worthy of a more widespread following and is to be encouraged.

In the view of venereologists, as revealed by a recent survey, less than a quarter of local authorities appear to treat seriously their obligations in prevention. The recent Newsom report on education offers an opportunity to fulfil these obligations in the schools. The relevant recommendation, now accepted by the Ministry of Education, reads as follows:

Positive guidance to adolescent boys and girls on sexual behaviour in general is essential. This should include biological, moral, social and personal aspects. Advice to parents on the physical and emotional problems of adolescents should be easily available. Schools, of whatever type, should provide opportunities for boys and girls to mix socially in a healthful and educative environment.

In addition the usefulness of various other forms of public education about the venereal diseases is recognized. Television, radio, short films, books and discussion groups all have a part to play. Integration of efforts should be helpful. For example, television programmes on the subject may be complemented by Local Authority endeavours.

Sexually transmitted diseases, whether labelled venereal or not, are in a sense among the most preventable. They are also among the most readily curable. They are dwarfed as a health problem by such questions as cancer, rheumatism and accidents. It is for these reasons that anti-V.D. propaganda and health and sex education are limited in their value and perhaps less effective than they were during war-time. The indications are that a resurgence of effort in educating the public is needed. Prosperity primarily dictates the present high and rising incidences of venereal disease in many countries. Its continuance in Britain must therefore lead us to anticipate new and high levels of infection. If we seriously wish to contain the situation within manageable bounds then the need for health education can be seen as an urgent necessity.

While this side of the problem and the sustained efforts of venereologists require constant survey, it is essentially the general social situation that clamours for resolution. Laird[66] says, 'the ultimate control of venereal disease lies outside the direct influence of the venereologist and will be both slow and difficult to achieve.' General social influences and efforts, whether in the socio-economic, moral or legal spheres, while by no means conducive to optimism, do not leave us completely devoid of a modicum of hope. What we can now clearly see is that in some degree venereal diseases are an indicator of social sickness. Perhaps this realization will bring us to a state of social awareness, somewhat pointedly depicted by Lord Caradon,[69] the U.K. representative at the United Nations, thus: '. . . we in our affluence become so soft, selfish, self-centred, superior and supercilious'. A sense of community conscience could eventually lead to action, and so to a more competent social structure.

What can medicine contribute?

Some of medicine's most notable achievements have been in the mastering of communicable diseases. Syphilitic and gono-coccal infections, however, remain the twin anachronisms of the scientific era in medicine. There are many reasons for this. When the diseases flourish, research tends to concentrate on problems of diagnosis and treatment, while between epidemics there is no stimulus to provide the impetus for fundamental research. Furthermore, earlier beliefs that penicillin would effect control at some irreducible and stable low level – the term 'dying diseases' was current in the 1950s – have proved to be unjustified. The same may be said for campaigns broadly based on education, prompt treatment, follow-up and contact tracing. Dr Brown, head of the Venereal Diseases Section of the United States Public Health Service, when referring to the closing of clinics and the cutting back of financial appropriations for the venereal diseases service, as happened in America in the 1950s, pointed out that the success of a campaign is likely to lead to the disappearance of the campaign rather than the disappearance of the disease.

Not the least of the reasons for failing to deal as effectively with the venereal diseases as we have done with, say, diphtheria or poliomyelitis has been the confusion of medicine and morals. In a vital passage in the British Medical Association's report on *Venereal Disease and Young People*[106] we read '. . . we believe [venereal disease] to be primarily a moral and social problem' and 'even if venereal diseases could be eliminated by medical means the social problems would still exist'. Here is an in-triguing idea. If we are unable to control men as individuals or societies, could we control, to the point of eradication, his venereal diseases?

At a meeting of the Medical Society for the Study of Venereal

Diseases in London in April 1958[75] there was a discussion on the
waning efficacy of penicillin in the treatment of gonorrhoea. It
was then contended that the aim should not be the modest one
of controlling the disease but outright eradication. This should
be sought through fundamental research calculated to produce a
prophylactic substance, for prevention by inoculation. It must be
said straight away that the outlook for any successful development of an immuno-prophylactic substance is not good.
Success may well depend on the discovery of some new concept
in bacteriology. Neither gonorrhoea nor syphilis is a disease in
which one attack confers a high degree of immunity. Why this
should be so is not known. It may be that the toxins, or poisons
produced by the organisms, are weak or only locally effective in
stimulating the production of antibodies, or that the organisms
favour sites relatively inaccessible to antibodies. These two
views would go some way to explain the self-limiting nature of
untreated gonorrhoea, so obvious in days gone by, and the
chronicity of syphilis in some people.

A curative type of vaccine was at one time in use for gonorrhoea. It was of little value. To date the gonococcus remains one
of the most neglected of organisms. One immediate drawback
to its study by the experimental worker is that no animal has
been found susceptible to it. It is, however, sixty years since any
reported attempt in this direction. In the meantime a lot has
been learned about tissue immunity and how it can be broken
down experimentally in the laboratory animal.

Suggestions made in 1958 regarding the detection of traces of
antibodies and the study of chemical constituents of the gonococcus have received little attention. The neglect afforded the
organism in the first half of the century largely continues.

Hope for the future comes from the W.H.O. Expert Committee Report on Gonococcal Infections,[118] which shows the
forms of organization and research needed to meet the present
crisis. In trying to offset 'the failure of control', the report makes
ten recommendations for improving diagnosis, public health
work and laboratory facilities. The laboratory research recommendations are clear and unequivocal. One of them calls for

coordinated efforts which might lead to definition of an immuno-prophylactic agent.

Super-infection of an already syphilitic person is rare. When a syphilitic has been treated adequately he is less likely to be infected artificially in experiments than is a person who has never had syphilis, according to research on volunteers in Sing-Sing Prison in the U.S.A. That childhood yaws may confer some degree of immunity to syphilis has already been mentioned. A faint promise of successful immunization may be implicit in these observations.

The idea of work in this direction has met with serious consideration by four or five experimental syphilologists in America. There has been a call for planned research. Dr John Knox, speaking at a seminar in Denver in January 1965, gave it as his considered opinion that if as much money was put into syphilis research as went into research on poliomyelitis – which did not kill or cripple as many people – a vaccine could be found in a few years.

Still further in the future, and even more highly speculative, are the possibilities for preventing other sexually transmitted diseases, especially non-specific urethritis, should its possibly viral origin be confirmed.

The proposed biological prevention of the venereal diseases would stand a fair chance of success. In no disease is it found necessary to inoculate 100 per cent of the potential victims to expect virtual eradication of the condition. Venereal diseases, which so typically afflict well-recognized groups, offer a situation which gives some hopes of success. Effective immunization, if and when it becomes available, would therefore be reserved in the first instance for prostitutes, those acquiring repeated infections and perhaps military personnel in time of war. There is, of course, nothing novel in the idea of vaccination or inoculation to prevent communicable disease. As a solitary weapon it has had some remarkable success, for example in diphtheria. This is in sharp contrast to the part played by treatment alone, which has not eradicated any common infection. In other diseases social measures combined with treatment have been only modestly effective, for example in dysentery. In the fight against tuberculosis it is the combination, and simultaneous pursuit, of social efforts, treatment and preventive inoculation which offers hopes of world-wide control to the point of eradication.

The venereal diseases show no tendency to yield to our best concerted legal, moral, psychological, sociological, political or religious efforts. Nor do the contributions of medical science to their treatment give help to any notable degree. The addition of a prophylactic approach, with its commendable array of precedents, merits our earliest attention. Without it, hopes of solving the enigma look like being denied to us.

References

1. AMBROSE, S. S. and TAYLOR, W. W., 'Study of etiology, epidemiology, and therapeusis of nongonococcal urethritis'. *American Journal of Syphilology*, 1953, 37, p. 501.

2. ASTRUC, J., *A Treatise of Venereal Diseases*. Translated by W. Barrowby, London, 1737.

3. BEVERIDGE, M. M., 'Social factors in male gonococcal infections'. *Public Health*, 1964, 78, p. 268.

4. BOTZOV, P., 'Epidemiology of gonorrhoea in Bulgaria'. *British Journal of Venereal Diseases*, 1961, 37, p. 132.

5. BOYD, J. T., CSONKA, G. W., and OATES, J. K., 'Epidemiology of non-specific urethritis'. *British Journal of Venereal Diseases*, 1958, 34, p. 40.

6. British Co-operative Clinical Group Study. *British Journal of Venereal Diseases*, 1956, 32, p. 21.

7. British Co-operative Clinical Group Study. *British Journal of Venereal Diseases*. 1960, 36, p. 216.

8. British Co-operative Clinical Group Study. *British Journal of Venereal Diseases*. 1962, 38, p. 1.

9. 'British Co-operative Clinical Group Gonorrhoea Study 1962'. *British Journal of Venereal Diseases*, 1963, 39, p. 149.

10. BURCH, T. A., REES, C. W., and REARDON, L. V., 'Epidemiological studies on human trichomoniasis'. *American Journal of Tropical Medicine and Hygiene*, 1959, 8, p. 312.

11. BURGESS, J. A., 'Trichomonas vaginalis infection from splashing in water closets'. *British Journal of Venereal Diseases*, 1963, 39, p. 248.

12. BUXTON, C. L., WEINMAN, D., and JOHNSON, O., 'Epidemiology of trichomonas vaginalis vaginitis: a progress report'. *Obstetrics and Gynaecology*, 1958, 12, p. 699.

13. CAMPBELL, D. J., quoted by GUTHE, T., 'Prevention of venereal infection'. *Bulletin of the World Health Organization*, 1958, 19, p. 416.

14. CAPINSKI, T. Z. and BACHURZEWSKI, J., 'Epidemiology and control of gonorrhoea in Poland'. *British Journal of Venereal Diseases*, 1961, 37, p. 100.

15. CARPENTER, C. M., 'Gonococcal resistance to penicillin in the light of recent literature'. *Bulletin of the World Health Organization*, 1961, 24, p. 321.

16. CATTERALL, R. D., 'Anorectal gonorrhoea'. *Proceedings of the Royal Society of Medicine*, 1962, 55, p. 871.

17. CATTERALL, R. D. and NICOL, C. S., 'Is trichomonal infestation a venereal disease?' *British Medical Journal*, 1960, 1, p. 1177.

18. *Census 1961 England and Wales*. Birth place and Nationality table. H.M.S.O.

19. COLLART, P., BOREL, L.-J., and DUREL, P., 'Significance of spiral organisms found after treatment in late human and experimental syphilis'. *British Journal of Venereal Diseases*, 1964, 40, p. 81.

20. CURJAL, H. E. B., 'An analysis of the human reasons underlying the failure to use a condom in 723 cases of venereal disease'. *Journal of the Royal Naval Medical Service*, 1964, 1, p. 203.

21. CURTIS, F. R. and WILKINSON, A. E., 'Sensitivity of gonococci to penicillin'. *British Journal of Venereal Diseases*, 1958, 34, p. 70.

22. DALZELL-WARD, A. J., NICOL, C. S., and HAWORTH, M. C., 'Group discussion with male venereal disease patients'. *British Journal of Venereal Diseases*, 1960, 36, p. 106.

23. DEVLIN, P. A. (Baron Devlin), *The Enforcement of Morals*. Oxford University Press, 1965.

24. DUNLOP, E. M. C., 'Epidemiology of gonorrhoea'. *British Journal of Venereal Diseases*, 1963, 39, p. 109.

25. Editorial. 'Infection of the eye and the genital tract by Tric virus'. *British Journal of Venereal Diseases*, 1964, 40, p. 1.

26. ELLISON, MARY, *Missing from Home*. Pan Books, London, 1964.

27. EPTON, NINA, *Love and the English*. Penguin Books, 1964.

28. FEO, L. G., 'The incidence of trichomonas vaginalis in the various age groups'. *American Journal of Tropical Medicine and Hygiene*, 1956, 5, p. 786.

29. FEO, L. G., VARANO, N. R., and FETTER, T. R., 'Trichomonas vaginalis in urethritis of the male'. *British Journal of Venereal Diseases*, 1956, 32, p. 233.

30. FESSLER, A., 'Advertisements in the treatment of venereal disease and the social history of venereal disease'. *British Journal of Venereal Diseases*, 1949, 25, p. 84.

31. FRENCH, ELEANOR, 'Prostitution'. *British Journal of Venereal Diseases*, 1955, 31, p. 113.

32. GARTMANN, E. and LEIBOVITZ, A., 'A study of non-gonococcal urethritis presumably venereal in origin, based on 588 infections in 529 patients'. *British Journal of Venereal Diseases*, 1955, 31, p. 92.

33. GASPARI, M., 'La prostitution en Italie', *Revue internationale de police criminelle*, No. 134, January 1960.

34. GIBBENS, T. C. N. and SILBERMAN, M., 'The clients of prostitutes'. *British Journal of Venereal Diseases*, 1960, 36, p. 113.

35. GISSLEN, H., HELLGREN, L., and STARCK, V., 'Incidence, age distribution and complications of gonorrhoea in Sweden'. *Bulletin of the World Health Organization*, 1961, 24, p. 367.

36. GJESTLAND, T., 'Oslo study of untreated syphilis; epidemiological investigation of natural course of syphilitic infection based upon re-study of Boeck–Bruusgaard material'. *Acta dermatologica and venereclogica* (Stockholm), 1955, 35, supplement p. 34.

37. GREEN, M. and MOORE, S., 'The homosexual in the V.D. clinic'. *British Journal of Venereal Diseases*, 1964, 40, p. 135.

38. GURR, C. E., *Modern School Girls*. Middlesex County Council.

39. GUTHE, T., 'The treponematoses as a world problem'. *British Journal of Venereal Diseases*, 1960, 34, p. 67.

40. GUTHE, T., 'Failure to control gonorrhoea'. *Bulletin of the World Health Organization*, 1961, 24, p. 297.

41. GUTHE, T., 'Prevention of venereal infection'. *Bulletin of the World Health Organization*, 1958, 19, p. 405.

42. HACKETT, C. J., 'Origin of treponematoses'. *Bulletin of the World Health Organization*, 1963, 29, p. 7.

43. HALL, T. ST. E., 'West Indians in Great Britain'. *British Journal of Venereal Diseases*, 1957, 33, p. 157.

44. HAWORTH, M. C. and NICOL, C. S., 'Tracing the contacts of male patients with acute gonorrhoea'. *British Journal of Venereal Diseases*, 1954, 30, p. 36.

45. HOOKINGS, C. E. and GRAVES, L. M., 'Benzathine penicillin in control of gonorrhoea'. *British Journal of Venereal Diseases*, 1957, 33, p. 40.

46. HORNE, G. O., 'The contemporary defaulter in a V.D. clinic'. *British Journal of Venereal Diseases*, 1953, 29, p. 210.

47. HUDSON, E. H., 'Treponematoses and African slavery'. *British Journal of Venereal Diseases*, 1964, 40, p. 43.

48. JEFFERISS, F. J. G., 'Venereal disease and the homosexual'. *British Journal of Venereal Diseases*, 1956, 32, p. 17.

49. JENSEN, T., 'Rectal gonorrhoea in women'. *British Journal of Venereal Diseases*, 1953, 29, p. 222.

50. KALLMAN, F. J., 'Twin sibships and the study of male homosexuality'. *American Journal of Human Genetics*, 1952, 4, p. 136.

51. KALLMAN, F. J., 'Comparative twin studies of the genetic aspects of male homosexuality'. *Journal of Nervous and Mental Diseases*, 1952, 115, p. 283.

52. KEIGHLEY, ELIZABETH, 'Venereal Diseases in women prisoners'. *British Journal of Venereal Diseases*, 1957, 33, p. 105.

53. KEIGHLEY, ELIZABETH, 'Trichomoniasis in a closed community: 100 per cent follow up'. *British Medical Journal*, 1962, 1, p. 95.

54. KEIGHLEY, ELIZABETH, 'Immaturity and venereal disease in teenage girls'. *British Journal of Venereal Diseases*, 1963, 39, p. 278.

55. KING, A. J., *Recent Advances in Venereology*. Churchill, London, 1964, p. 367, 477.

56. KING, A. J., 'These Dying Diseases: Venereology in Decline?' *Lancet*, 1958, 1, p. 651.

57. KING, A. J., 'For and against treatment before diagnosis'. *British Journal of Venereal Diseases*, 1954, 30, p. 13.

58. KING, A. J. and NICOL, C. S., *Venereal Diseases*. Cassell, London, 1964, p. 210.

59. KINSEY, A. C., POMEROY, W. B., and MARTIN, C. E., *Sex Behaviour in the Human Male*. W. B. Saunders & Co., Philadelphia and London, 1948.

60. KITE, E. DE C. and GRIMBLE, A., 'Psychiatric aspects of venereal disease'. *British Journal of Venereal Diseases*, 1963, 39, p. 173.

61. KNIGHT, G., 'Results of the treatment of gonorrhoea in the Birmingham clinic'. *British Journal of Venereal Diseases*, 1958, 34, p. 223.

62. KOMOROWSKA, A., KURNATOWSKA, A., and LINIECKA, J., 'Presence of trichomonas vaginalis in girls depending on hygienic conditions'. *Journal Polish Towarzystwo, Parazytologiozne*, 1962, 8, p. 247.

63. LAIRD, S. M., 'Defence Regulation 33 B'. *Journal of the Royal Sanitary Institute*, 1946, 66, p. 193.

64. LAIRD, S. M., 'Elimination of congenital syphilis'. *British Journal of Venereal Diseases*, 1959, 35, p. 15.

65. LAIRD, S. M., 'Incidence of General Paralysis of the Insane'. *British Medical Journal*, 1962, 1, p. 524.

66. LAIRD, S. M., 'Figures and fancies'. *British Journal of Venereal Diseases*, 1958, 34, p. 137.

67. LAIRD, S. M. and MORTON, R. S., 'The ecology and control of gonorrhoea'. *British Journal of Venereal Diseases*, 1959, 35, p. 187.

68. LAIRD, S. M., *Venereal Disease in Britain*. Penguin Books, 1943.

69. LORD CARADON, report in the *Daily Telegraph*, 24 December 1964.

70. MACFARLANE, W. V., 'Prevention of congenital syphilis'. *Lancet*, 1950, 1, p. 1069.

71. MACFARLANE, W. V., SWAN, W. G. A., and ERVINE, R. E., 'Cardiovascular disease in syphilis'. *British Medical Journal*, 1956, 1, p. 827.

72. MCELLIGOTT, G. L. M., 'Venereal disease and the public health'. *British Medical Journal*, 1960, 36, p. 207.

73. MORTON, R. S. and READ, L., 'Non-gonococcal urethritis'. *British Journal of Venereal Diseases*, 1957, 33, p. 223.

74. MORTON, R. S., 'The precontemporary syphilitic defaulter'. *British Journal of Venereal Diseases*, 1954, 30, p. 198.

75. MORTON, R. S., 'Sensitivity of gonococci to penicillin'. *British Journal of Venereal Diseases*, 1958, 34, p. 81.

76. MORTON, R. S., 'Some aspects of the early history of syphilis in Scotland'. *British Journal of Venereal Diseases*, 1962, 38, p. 175.

77. NELSON, R. A., and MEYER, M. M., 'Immobilization of treponema pallidum in vitro by antibody produced in syphilitic infection'. *Journal of Experimental Medicine*, 1949, 89, p. 369.

78. NIELSEN, I. S., 'Gonorrhoea in teenagers'. *British Journal of Venereal Diseases*, 1961, 37, p. 138.

79. NICOL, C. S., 'Diagnosis of trichomonal vaginalis urethritis in the male as a routine clinic procedure'. *British Journal of Venereal Diseases*, 1958, 34, p. 192.

80. NICOL, C. S., 'Venereal diseases – moral standards and public opinion'. *British Journal of Venereal Diseases*, 1963, 39, p. 168.

81. NICOL, C. S., Report: British Federation against the Venereal Diseases. *British Journal of Venereal Diseases*, 1958, 34, p. 124.

82. OATES, J. K., 'Role of the prostate in non-specific urethritis'. *Acta dermatologica–venereologica* (Stockholm). Proceedings 11th International Congress in Dermatology 1957, volume 3, p. 994.

83. O'HARE, J., 'The road to promiscuity'. *British Journal of Venereal Diseases*, 1960, 36, p. 122.

84. PARKIN, E. and STENGEL, E., 'Incidence of suicide attempts in an urban community'. *British Medical Journal*, 1965, 2, p. 133.

85. PETER, R., *Les infestations avec trichomonas*. Masson, Paris, 1957, p. 155.

86. PONTING, L. I., 'Social aspects of venereal diseases in young people in Leeds and London'. *British Journal of Venereal Diseases*, 1963, 39, p. 273.

87. Public Health Report. *World Forum on Syphilis*. U.S. Public Health Service, Washington D.C., 1963, 78, p. 295.

88. Report of the Chief Medical Officer for 1962: *On the State of the Public Health*. H.M.S.O., 1963, pp. 64 and 233. S.O. Code pp. 32–518.

89. Report of the Chief Medical Officer for 1963: *On the State of the Public Health*. H.M.S.O., 1964. Part II, p. 67.

90. Report of the Chief Medical Officer for 1957: *On the State of the Public Health*. H.M.S.O., 1958, p. 282.

91. Report of Conference: 'Tomorrow's Parents'. *British Medical Journal*, 1964, 2, p. 1260.

92. ROSEDALE, N., 'Female consorts of men with non-gonococcal urethritis'. *British Journal of Venereal Diseases*, 1959, 35, p. 245.

93. ROSHAHN, P. D., 'The adverse influence of syphilitic injections on the longevity of mice and men'. *Archives of Dermatology and Syphilis*, Chicago, 1952, 66, p. 547.

94. SCHMIDT, H., HAUGE, L., and SCHØNNING, L., 'Incidence of homosexuals among syphilitics'. *British Journal of Venereal Diseases*, 1963, 39, p. 264.

95. SCHOFIELD, M., *The Sexual Behaviour of Young People*. Longmans, 1965.

96. SHAFER, J. K., USILTON, L. T., and GLESSON, G. A., 'Untreated syphilis in the male Negro'. Public Health Report, Washington, 1954, 69, p. 684.

97. SHAW, H. N., HENRIKSER, V., KESSEL, J. F., and THOMPSON, C. F., 'Clinical and laboratory evaluation of "vagisol" in treatment of trichomonas vaginalis vaginitis'. *Western Journal of Surgery*, 1952, 60, p. 563.

98. SEQUEIRA, P. J. L., 'Serology of the venereal diseases'. *British Journal of Venereal Diseases*, 1962, 38, p. 9.

99. STENGEL, E., *Suicide and Attempted Suicide*. Pelican Books, 1964.

100. *The Venereal Diseases*. Office of Health Economics, London, 1963.

101. THOMAS, E. W., SHAFER, J. K., and ZWALLY, M. R., 'Factors leading to development of late manifestations of syphilis'. *American Journal of Syphilis*, 1954, 38, p. 531.

102. 'Treatment of Venereal Diseases outside the Hospital Service'. *British Journal of Venereal Diseases*, 1959, 35, p. 111.

103. TRUSSELL, R. E., *Trichmonas Vaginalis and Trichomoniasis*. Thomas Springfield, Illinois, 1947.

104. UNITED STATES DEPARTMENT OF HEALTH AND WELFARE. PUBLIC HEALTH SERVICE. *The Eradication of Syphilis*. Public Health Service Publication, 1962, 918, p. 13.

105. UNWIN, J. C., *Sex and Culture*. Oxford University Press, 1934.

106. *Venereal Diseases and Young People*. A British Medical Association Report, 1964.

107. VERHEYE, H., 'Contribution à l'étude des infections à Trichomonas vaginalis en rapport avec le pH vaginal chez la Congolaise'. (Relation of trichomonas vaginalis infections to the vaginal pH of the native Congo woman.) *Ann. Soc. Belge Médecine Tropique*, 1956, 36, p. 499.

108. WANG, T. K. and HSIA, T. F., 'Treatment of trichomonas vaginalis infections with plant germicides and medicinal herbs'. *Chinese Medical Journal*, 1958, 77, p. 363.

109. WATSON, CICELY, 'Recent changes in French policy on venereal disease and prostitution'. *British Journal of Venereal Diseases*, 1954, 30, p. 203.

110. WATT, L., 'Venereal diseases in adolescents'. *British Medical Journal*, 1964, 2, p. 858.

111. WEST, D. J., *Homosexuality*. Pelican Books, 1963.

112. WHITTINGTON, M. J., 'The incidence of trichomonas vaginalis in a sample of the general population'. *Journal of Obstetrics and Gynaecology of the British Empire*, 1951, 58, p. 299.

113. WHITTINGTON, M. J., 'Epidemiology of infections with trichomonas vaginalis in the light of improved diagnostic methods'. *British Journal of Venereal Diseases*, 1957, 33, p. 80.

114. WILLCOX, R. R., 'Prostitution and venereal disease'. *British Journal of Venereal Diseases*, 1962, 38, p. 37.

115. WILLCOX, R. R., 'Age group and country of origin of cases of gonorrhoea in England and Wales'. *British Journal of Venereal Diseases*, 1963, 39, p. 214.

116. WILLCOX, R. R., 'Treatment before diagnosis in venereology'. *British Journal of Venereal Diseases*, 1954, 30, p. 7.

117. WORLD HEALTH ORGANIZATION, Technical Report No. 190: 'Expert Committee on Venereal Infections and Treponematosis'. (Fifth Report) Geneva, 1960.

118. WORLD HEALTH ORGANIZATION, Technical Report No. 262. 'Expert Committee on Gonococcal Infections'. (First Report) Geneva, 1963.

119. WORLD HEALTH ORGANIZATION, *Chronicle*, 1964, 18, p. 48.

120. WORLD HEALTH ORGANIZATION, 'British Co-operative Clinical Group. Syphilis in first year of infection, Country of Origin Study'. WHO/VDT/325 dated 5 October 1964.

Index

Ages of infected, 114, 116
Alcohol, 131, 138
Anatomy, 51, 55
Anti-social behaviour, 113, 164
Ante-natal blood tests, 38
Anxiety, 48, 109
Antibiotics, 63, 154
Arthritis, 58, 98, 160
Astruc, 27
'At risk' groups: see Young people, Immigration, Homosexuality and Itinerants.
Attitudes to V.D., 13

Balanitis, 109
Bartholinitis, 53
Bell, Benjamin, 21
Blood tests for syphilis, 38, 76, 87, 141, 150
Blindness, 58, 83, 160
British Federation Against V.D., 136
Bulgaria, 35

Central Council for Health Education, 135
Chancroid, 16, 29, 44, 65
Clinics: see Special clinics
'Cluster' testing, 147
'Cold sores': see Herpes

Columbian theory of origin of syphilis, 22
Commonwealth Immigrants Act, 127, 163
Compulsory treatment, 30–31
Contact tracing, 141
Condoms, 138
Costs, 32
'Contact slip', 142

Deaths, 43, 81, 84, 160
Denmark, 36, 41, 116
Delinquency, 113, 165
Diagnosis, problems of, 149–50
Divorce, 140, 145

Education, public, 135, 169
Epidemiological treatment, 155

Follow-up examination, problems of, 157
France, 41, 120
Fungus: see Moniliasis

Girls, 58, 106, 115, 164
Gonorrhoea, 16, 20, 33, 37, 50
    asymptomatic, 53, 56, 57
    complications, female, 53, 58, 160
    complications, male, 56, 58, 160
    diagnostic methods, 59, 149
    neonatal, 58

Gonorrhea (*continued*)
  rectal, 54, 57
  treatment, 63, 153

Health visitor, 143
Herpes, of genitals, 109
History, 19
Homosexuality, 57, 71, 128, 156, 163

Illegitimacy, 113, 166
Immaturity, 118
Immigration, 124, 163
Incubation periods, 53, 56, 70
Information on V.D., 110
Infectious diseases, 39, 43
Italy, 120
Itinerants, 128

Juvenile delinquency: *see* Delinquency

Law and legal considerations, 31,
  121, 127, 140–41, 145, 163
Lice, 108
Lymphogranuloma venereum, 16,
  44, 65

Marriage, 140, 144
Mortality: *see* Deaths
Mercury, 28
Moniliasis, 108

Non-gonococcal urethritis, 45, 91,
  104
Non-specific urethritis, 17, 93, 151
  complications, 95, 98
  consideration of possible causes,
    94
  recurrence, 97
  treatment of, 97
  and the female consort, 99

Parents, 168
Patients, number of, 47, 110
Penicillin, 63, 87, 151, 154

Poland, 35
Prevention, 135, 138, 171
Prosperity, 112, 133, 169
Promiscuity, 117, 126, 143, 166
Prostatitis, 57, 96
Prostitution, 119, 166
Public health, 135, 141

Rectal gonorrhoea, 53, 57
Rectal syphilis, 70
Running away from home, 165
Reiter's disease or syndrome, 98

Salpingitis, 54
Scabies, 108
Sex contacts, 98, 107, 141, 152
Sex education: *see* Education
Sexually transmitted disease, 15, 17,
  91
Social class, 114
Social history, 29
Social aspects, 29, 112, 162, 167
Special clinics, 47
Sterility, 57
Suicide, 166
Sweden, 41
Syphilis, 16, 22, 38, 40, 68
  and pregnancy, 38, 84
  congenital, 70, 84
  diagnosis, 68, 72–3, 75, 76
  latent, 67, 74
  late, 79
  primary, 70
  secondary, 72
  treatment of, 87
  without treatment, 72, 74, 86,
    160
Spirochaeta pallida: *see* Treponema
  pallidum

Tracing of infected contacts: *see*
  Contact tracing
Treatment problems, 151
Treponema pallidum, 68, 152

Treponematosis (and treponema-
   toses), 26, 89
Trichomoniasis, 17, 46, 100, 151
Thrush: *see* Moniliasis

Unitarian theory of origin of
   syphilis, 24
U.S.A., 33, 41, 147

U.S.S.R., 35, 132

Vaginal thrush: *see* Moniliasis

Warts, 108

Yaws, 26, 43, 89
Young people, 115, 168

More About Penguins and Pelicans

If you have enjoyed reading this book you may wish to know that *Penguin Book News* appears every month. It is an attractively illustrated magazine containing a complete list of books published by Penguins and still in print, together with details of the month's new books. A specimen copy will be sent free on request.

Penguin Book News is obtainable from most bookshops; but you may prefer to become a regular subscriber at 3s. for twelve issues. Just write to Dept. EP, Penguin Books Ltd, Harmondsworth, Middlesex, enclosing a cheque or postal order, and you will be put on the mailing list.

Some other books published by Penguins are described on the following pages.

Note: *Penguin Book News* is not available in the U.S.A., Canada or Australia.

Alcoholism

Niel Kessel and Henry Walton

Alcoholism is a serious illness. Physically it damages the body and shortens life. Socially it causes untold harm not only to the sufferer but also to his family.

Although middle-aged men are most affected, women alcoholics are increasing in number and young alcoholics are becoming numerous.

This book begins by considering what distinguishes the excessive from the social drinker. Physical, psychological and social factors all influence the development of the condition. What are alcoholics like and what are their chances of recovery? What part should the family and friends play, and the doctor and the hospitals? What can be learned from Alcoholics Anonymous?

Alcoholism is a fascinating study designed to explore, from the standpoint of the general reader, these aspects of an important social and medical problem.

The Psychology of Sex

Oswald Schwarz

As morality is the principle which governs and guards any human relationship, the main theme of this book is an analysis of the interaction of the physical sexual urge and the moral principle, with the conclusion that nothing that is truly natural can be really immoral. Such a statement makes sense only if morality is properly defined and clearly distinguished from what one may call conventional taboos. The much-discussed 'problem of sex' then stands revealed as the result of confusion of the real or essential morality with time-honoured but outworn convention.

On this basis the author analyses the various forms of sexual activity: masturbation, homosexuality in youth, prostitution, 'affairs'; and demonstrates that they are stages in a development which ultimately leads to marriage as the complete form of sexual relationship. A few case histories serve to illustrate the basic theory of this book and its application. The thesis that an 'essentially' moral sex life is the expression of the whole personality throws a light on, and provides a scientific basis for the discussion of, some social aspects of sex life, such as prostitution, birth control, and divorce.

The Physiology of Sex

Kenneth Walker

Popular works on sex have appeared in large numbers in recent years: very few of them have treated the subject from all its aspects, physiological, emotional, and social, in a way which combines the imparting of the necessary information with a spirit of helpfulness.

Kenneth Walker provides a clear, straightforward statement of the facts of sex and its problems in the life of the individual and the community. He writes strictly as a scientist for adult readers, and he refrains from passing judgement, but he confesses his own belief that the questions raised cannot be satisfactorily answered in a world that is empty of spiritual values.

'Mr Walker's treatment of the subject is thorough and complete. Everything that you can find in Havelock Ellis, Bertrand Russell, or their American equivalents, you will find treated very honestly and fully in this little book. . . . His book shirks nothing, and every opinion that he expresses is candid and straightforward' – *The New Generation*.

Crime in a Changing Society

Howard Jones

Throughout the Western world crime is on the increase:
in America four serious crimes are committed every minute
and in Britain the number of people involved in crime has
more than doubled since the 1930s. The causes and treatment
of criminal behaviour are now of urgent interest to the man
in the street, and it is for him that Dr Jones has written
Crime in a Changing Society. It is the first general survey
of the history, methods, and aims of criminology and
penology to have been aimed specifically at the general
reader.

The discussion ranges from 'criminal areas', the psychology
of abnormal offenders and the influences of heredity and
intelligence to the 'punishment versus treatment' debate, the
structure of penal reform, and the meaning of teenage
violence.

Here is both a simple, concise account of the crime problem
and a social critique of the relation of criminal behaviour to
patterns of social change in contemporary Britain.